NCLEX-PN

250 New-Format Questions

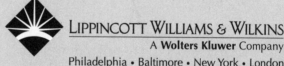

LIPPINCOTT WILLIAMS & WILKINS
A **Wolters Kluwer** Company

Philadelphia • Baltimore • New York • London
Buenos Aires • Hong Kong • Sydney • Tokyo

STAFF

Publisher
Judith A. Schilling McCann, RN, MSN

Editorial Director
David Moreau

Clinical Director
Joan M. Robinson, RN, MSN

Senior Art Director
Arlene Putterman

Editors
Jaime L. Stockslager (senior editor), Tracy S. Diehl
(senior associate editor), Kevin Haworth,
Barbara Hodgson, Brenna H. Mayer, Liz Schaeffer,
Pam Wingrod

Clinical Editors
Marcy Caplin, RN, MSN; Collette Hendler, RN, BS, CCRN;
Beverly Ann Tscheschlog, RN, BSN

Copy Editor
Kimberly Bilotta

Designer
Debra Moloshok (project manager)

Digital Composition Services
Diane Paluba (manager), Joyce Rossi Biletz (senior
desktop assistant), Donna S. Morris (senior desktop
assistant

Manufacturing
Patricia K. Dorshaw (senior manager), Beth Janae Orr
(book production coordinator)

Editorial Assistants
Megan Lane Aldinger, Tara Carter-Bell,
Arlene P. Claffee, Linda Ruhf

The clinical treatments described and recommended in this publication are based on research and consultation with nursing, medical, and legal authorities. To the best of our knowledge, these procedures reflect currently accepted practice. Nevertheless, they can't be considered absolute and universal recommendations. For individual applications, all recommendations must be considered in light of the patient's clinical condition and, before administration of new or infrequently used drugs, in light of the latest package-insert information. The authors and publisher disclaim any responsibility for any adverse effects resulting from the suggested procedures, from any undetected errors, or from the reader's misunderstanding of the text.

PN250 — D N O
05 04   10 9 8 7 6 5 4 3

Library of Congress Cataloging-in-Publication Data

NCLEX-PN 250 new-format questions : preparing for the revised NCLEX-PN.
    p. ; cm.
    1. Practical nursing — Examinations, questions, etc. 2. Practical nursing — Outlines, syllabi, etc. 3. Practical nurses — Licenses — United States — Examinations — Study guides.
    [DNLM: 1. Nursing, Practical — Examination Questions. 2. Nursing Care — Examination Questions. WY 18.2 N3368 2004] I. Title: NCLEX-PN two hundred fifty new-format questions. II. Lippincott Williams & Wilkins.

RT55.N415 2004
610.73'06'93076 — dc21
ISBN 1-58255-308-4 (alk. paper)   2003013189

Contents

Contributors

Julie Akins, RN, BSN
Assistant Professor, Practical Nursing
College of Southern Idaho
Twin Falls

Ann Carmack, RN, MSN
Consultant
Kearney, Mo.

Linda P. Finch, RN, PhD
Assistant Professor
Loewenberg School of Nursing
University of Memphis

Bobbie L. Hunter, RN, MSN, CFNP
Nursing Instructor
PN Program Manager
Columbus (Ga.) Technical College

Karla Jones, RN, MS
Nursing Faculty
Treasure Valley Community College
Ontario, Ore.

Audrey Knippa, RN, MPH
Nursing Instructor
Clastop Community College
Astoria, Ore.

Sandra Liming, RN, MN, PhC
PN Program Coordinator
Instructor
North Seattle Community College

Dawna Martich, RN, MSN
Clinical Trainer
American Healthways
Pittsburgh, Pa.

Diana L. Rupert, RN,C, MSN
Faculty
Conemaugh School of Nursing
Johnstown, Pa.

Bruce Austin Scott, MSN, APRN, BC
Instructor
San Joaquin Delta College
Stockton, Calif.
Staff Nurse
University of California Davis Medical Center
Sacramento, Calif.

Catherine Shields, RN, BSN
Practical Nursing Instructor
Career and Technical Institute School of Nursing
Lakehurst, N.J.

Linda S. Wood, RN, MSN
Director of Practical Nursing
Massanutten Technical Center
Harrisonburg, Va.

Preface

You've worked hard to earn your degree. You're ready to move ahead in your career and begin your nursing practice. Only one thing stands in your way — the National Council Licensure Examination for Practical Nurses (NCLEX-PN). Every nursing student is familiar with the pressure and anxiety involved with taking the NCLEX-PN. As if the stress of the standard test questions weren't enough, however, the National Council of State Boards of Nursing (NCSBN) recently added three types of alternate item questions to the NCLEX. But don't worry, *NCLEX-PN: 250 New-Format Questions* is a cutting-edge review book that will help you become fully prepared for every type of question you may encounter on the NCLEX.

The first type of alternate item format is the multiple-response multiple-choice question. Unlike a traditional multiple-choice question, each multiple-response multiple-choice question has more than one correct answer, and it may contain more than four possible answer options. You'll recognize this type of question because you'll be asked to select **all** answers that apply — not just the **best** answer (as may be requested in the more traditional multiple-choice questions).

When you encounter one of these questions in this review book, read the question and all possible answers carefully. Place a check mark in the box next to all options that correctly answer the question. Keep in mind that, for each multiple-response multiple-choice question, you must select **at least two answers** and you must select **all correct answers** for the item to be counted as correct. On the NCLEX, there is no partial credit in the scoring of these items.

The second type of alternate item format is the fill-in-the-blank. These questions require you to provide the answer yourself, rather than select it from a list of options. For these questions, write your answer in the blank space provided after the question. Keep in mind that the computerized version of the NCLEX may require that you type in a very specific response in order for it to be considered correct (for example, "Mammography" rather than "Mammogram").

For purposes of this review, be as specific as possible with each of your answers to fill-in-the-blank questions. The answers we've supplied are the shortest, most precise responses, although, as noted above, variations may be possible. The NCSBN has not yet made clear how it will handle such variations on possible answers on its computerized test.

The third and final type of alternate item format is a question in which you will be asked to identify an area on an illustration or graphic. For these so-called "Hot spot" questions, the computerized exam will ask you to place your cursor over the correct area on an illustration.

When reviewing such questions in this book, read the question and then mark an X on the illustration in the left-hand column to indicate your answer. In the right-hand column, correct answers are similarly indicated by an X on the duplicate illustration. Try to be as precise as possible when marking the location. As with the fill-in-the-blanks, the identification questions on the computerized exam may require extremely precise answers in order for them to be considered correct.

These new alternate item formats are sure to make the NCLEX exam even more challenging than it has been in the past. Luckily, *NCLEX-PN: 250 New-Format Questions* was specifically developed to help you prepare for and excel at each of these types of questions. This helpful review book will boost your confidence and ease your anxiety.

A useful supplementary study guide, this book includes 250 alternate-format questions that cover all of the topics tested on the exam—including fundamentals of nursing, medical-surgical nursing, maternal-infant nursing, pediatric nursing, and psychiatric and mental health nursing. For each type of question, you'll find the correct answer as well as clear, concise rationales for correct and incorrect answers. You'll also find the associated nursing process step, client needs category and subcategory, and cognitive level.

The convenient two-column format (with questions on the left and answers on the right) enhances your preparation process by giving you instant feedback and saves you the time of flipping to the back of the book to find the correct answer.

The review questions provided in this book will test your knowledge base and improve your test-taking skills as well as help you become familiar with the format of the new questions. All of the questions were written by nurses and approximate the real questions you'll find on the NCLEX.

The NCSBN has not yet established a percentage of alternate item formats to be administered to each candidate. In fact, your exam may contain only one alternate item format. Be confident in knowing that the questions in this book cover relevant information in a challenging format that can be useful even if your NCLEX examination does not include these new format questions. Also, in your rush to prepare for the new format questions, don't forget to review practice questions that follow the standard four-option, multiple-choice format. These questions will still compose the bulk of the test.

Remember that the process of testing and introducing new alternate-format questions into the NCLEX is ongoing. Because the test format is subject to change, be sure to consult the "Testing services" section of the NCSBN web site (*www.ncsbn.org*) as your exam date nears for the most up-to-date information on the NCLEX.

You've been diligently preparing for this all-important exam for years. *NCLEX-PN: 250 New-Format Questions* is the next logical extension of that sound preparation, the final resource you need to meet the challenge of passing NCLEX and moving on to the rewards of your nursing career. Good luck.

Part 1

Fundamentals of nursing

1. The nurse is caring for a client who sustained a chemical burn in his right eye. She is preparing to irrigate the eye with sterile normal saline solution. Which steps are appropriate when performing the procedure?

Select all that apply:

☐ **A.** Tilt the client's head toward his left eye.

☐ **B.** Place absorbent pads in the area of the client's shoulder.

☐ **C.** Wash hands and put on gloves.

☐ **D.** Place the irrigation syringe directly on the cornea.

☐ **E.** Direct the solution onto the exposed conjunctival sac from the inner to outer canthus.

☐ **F.** Irrigate the eye for 1 minute.

ANSWER: B, C, E

Rationale: The nurse should place absorbent pads in the area of the shoulder to prevent saturating the client's clothing and bed linens. She should also wash her hands and put on gloves to reduce the transmission of microorganisms. The solution should be directed from the inner to outer canthus of the eye to prevent contamination of the unaffected eye. The head should be tilted toward the affected (right) eye to facilitate drainage and to prevent irrigating solution from entering the left eye. The irrigation syringe should be held about 1" (2.5 cm) above the eye to prevent injury to the cornea. In a chemical exposure, the eye should be irrigated for at least 10 minutes.

Nursing process step: Implementation

Client needs category: Physiological integrity

Client needs subcategory: Reduction of risk potential

Cognitive level: Application

2. The nurse is assigned to assist with caring for a client who has had a cardiac catheterization. She plans to keep the involved leg straight for the prescribed time and maintain bed rest. The nurse should not elevate the head of the bed greater than what number of degrees?

ANSWER: 30

Rationale: After cardiac catheterization, the nurse should elevate the head of the bed no more than 30 degrees in order to prevent arterial occlusion. In addition, the client should be maintained on bed rest and the extremity in which the catheter was inserted should be kept straight.

Nursing process step: Planning

Client needs category: Physiological integrity

Client needs subcategory: Reduction of risk potential

Cognitive level: Application

3. A nursing home resident is admitted to the hospital for evaluation and treatment of chronic diarrhea. The nurse plans to place the client on isolation precautions. Which type of isolation is most appropriate?

_____

ANSWER: Contact

Rationale: The purpose of isolation is to prevent the spread of infection to other clients. Contact isolation is normally used for GI infections and diarrhea. It is also used for wound infections with drainage or draining abscesses.

Nursing process step: Planning

Client needs category: Safe, effective care environment

Client needs subcategory: Safety and infection control

Cognitive level: Application

---

4. A hospitalized client asks the nurse for "something for pain." Which information is most important for the nurse to gather before administering the medication?

Select all that apply:

□ **A.** Administration time of the last dose

□ **B.** Client's pain level on a scale of 1 to 10

□ **C.** Type of medication the client has been taking

□ **D.** Beeper number of the client's physician

□ **E.** Client's most current height and weight

□ **F.** Effectiveness of prior dose of medication

ANSWER: A, B, C, F

Rationale: The nurse needs to know when the last dose was administered. Some clients request pain medication earlier than is ordered by the physician. Pain, the fifth vital sign, should be assessed using a pain scale and documented in the nursing notes whenever a pain medication is given. Pain is usually reassessed about 30 minutes after the medication is given. Physicians commonly order several different types of pain medication based on the client's condition. It is important for the nurse to know which medication and which route was used to administer prior dosages. Evaluating the effectiveness of medications is also an important nursing function when managing the client's pain. Therefore, she should ask the client if the prior dose was helpful. Knowing the beeper number of the client's physician is not as important as the other choices, although most nurses know the name of their clients' physicians. Most medications are ordered based on the client's weight and height. This information would have been obtained on admission.

Nursing process step: Data collection

Client needs category: Physiological integrity

Client needs subcategory: Basic care and comfort

Cognitive level: Application

5. The nurse is completing the intake and output record for a client who was restarted on his regular diet after being on nothing-by-mouth status for laboratory studies. The client has had the following intake and output during the shift:

Intake: 4 oz of cranberry juice, 1/2 cup of oat-meal, 2 slices of toast, 8 oz of black decaffeinated coffee, tuna fish sandwich, 1/2 cup of fruit-flavored gelatin, 1 cup of cream of mushroom soup, 6 oz. of 1% milk, 16 oz of water
Output: 1,300 ml of urine

How many milliliters should the nurse document as the client's intake?

ANSWER: 1,380

Rationale: There are 30 ml in each ounce and 240 ml in each cup. The fluid intake for this client includes 4 oz (120 ml) of cranberry juice, 8 oz (240 ml) of coffee, 1/2 cup (120 ml) of fruit-flavored gelatin, 1 cup (240 ml) of cream of mushroom soup, 6 oz (180 ml) of milk, and 16 oz (480 ml) of water, for a total of 1,380.

Nursing process step: Data collection

Client needs category: Physiological integrity

Client needs subcategory: Basic care and comfort

Cognitive level: Application

6. A client is ordered to receive a sodium phosphate enema for relief of constipation. Proper administration of the enema includes which of the following steps?

Select all that apply:

☐ **A.** Chill the solution by placing it in the refrigerator for 10 minutes.

☐ **B.** Assist the client into Sims' position.

☐ **C.** Wash hands and put on gloves.

☐ **D.** Insert the tip of the container 1/2" into the rectum.

☐ **E.** Allow gravity to instill the solution.

☐ **F.** Encourage the client to retain the solution for 5 to 15 minutes.

ANSWER: B, C, F

Rationale: To administer an enema, the nurse should place the client into Sims' position or a knee-chest position. Washing hands and putting on gloves is necessary to reduce the transmission of microorganisms. To promote the effectiveness of the enema, the nurse should encourage the client to retain the solution for at least 5 minutes. The solution should be warmed rather than chilled to promote comfort. To administer the solution effectively and deliver it to the appropriate location, the nurse should insert the full length of the tip into the rectum. The nurse should compress the container to deliver the solution under positive pressure and not by gravity.

Nursing process step: Implementation

Client needs category: Physiological integrity

Client needs subcategory: Basic care and comfort

Cognitive level: Application

7. A postoperative client has an abdominal incision. While getting out of bed, the client reports feeling a "pulling" sensation in his abdominal wound. The nurse assesses the client's wound and finds that it has separated and the abdominal organs are protruding. Which nursing interventions are most appropriate at this time?

Select all that apply:

☐ **A.** Notify the client's primary physician.

☐ **B.** Cover the wound with saline-soaked sterile gauze.

☐ **C.** Give the client a dose of antibiotics.

☐ **D.** Order an abdominal binder from the supply department.

☐ **E.** Push the organs back into the abdomen.

☐ **F.** Assess the client for signs of shock.

Rationale: Dehiscence (the separation of the surgical incision) and evisceration (the protruding of the abdominal organs) are considered medical emergencies. Therefore, the client's physician should be notified immediately and the nurse should prepare the client for surgery. While the nurse is waiting for the physician to arrive, the wound and the abdominal organs should be covered with saline-soaked sterile gauze. Saline is an isotonic solution that prevents damage to the client's tissue, and sterile gauze is used to prevent wound infection. Even though wound infection is the most common cause of dehiscence, administering antibiotics without a physician's order is not permissible and can result in the loss of a nursing license. An abdominal binder may be appropriate but only after the client returns from the operating room. Pushing the organs back into the abdomen is inappropriate and could result in rupture, hemorrhage, or strangulation of the bowel. Usually, dehiscence and evisceration produce little bleeding and, therefore, assessing for shock is not necessary at this time.

Nursing process step: Implementation

Client needs category: Physiological integrity

Client needs subcategory: Reduction of risk potential

Cognitive level: Analysis

---

8. A client comes to the facility complaining of flulike symptoms. The nurse plans to take the client's temperature orally, using a glass thermometer. What is the minimum number of minutes that the nurse should wait before removing the thermometer from the client's mouth and checking the temperature?

_____

Rationale: Three minutes is the minimum amount of time needed for accurate measurement of a client's oral temperature.

Nursing process step: Implementation

Client needs category: Physiological integrity

Client needs subcategory: Basic care and comfort

Cognitive level: Knowledge

9. A teenage boy suffers a broken leg as a result of a car accident and is taken to the emergency department. A plaster cast is applied. Before discharge, the nurse provides the client with instructions regarding cast care. Which instructions are most appropriate?

Select all that apply:

☐ **A.** Support the wet cast with pillows until it dries.

☐ **B.** Use a hair dryer to speed the drying process.

☐ **C.** Use the fingertips when moving the wet cast.

☐ **D.** Apply powder to the inside of the cast after it dries.

☐ **E.** Notify the physician if itching occurs under the cast.

☐ **F.** Avoid putting straws or hangers inside the cast.

ANSWER: A, F

Rationale: Supporting the wet cast with pillows prevents the cast from changing shape and interfering with the alignment of the fractured bone. The nurse should instruct the client not to place sharp objects, such as straws or hangers, down the inside of the cast to avoid the risk of impairing the skin and causing infection. Using a hair dryer is not advised because it dries the cast unevenly, can cause burns to the tissue, and can crack the cast, causing poor alignment to the injured bone. The palms, not the fingertips, should be used when handling the wet cast because fingertips can dent the cast, thus causing pressure points that can affect the skin's integrity. Powder should not be used because it can cake under the cast. Itching is a common occurrence with casts because the skin cells are unable to slough as they normally would and the dry skin causes itching. Normally, the physician is not called for this problem.

Nursing process step: Implementation

Client needs category: Physiological integrity

Client needs subcategory: Basic care and comfort

Cognitive level: Comprehension

10. The nurse investigates the smell of smoke in the hallway of the long-term care unit. She enters a client's room and finds that the wastebasket is on fire. The nurse takes immediate action based on the RACE mnemonic. According to this protocol, what is the first priority?

ANSWER: Rescue

Rationale: RACE sets priority actions in the event of a fire. RACE stands for:

    R – Rescue
    A – Alarm
    C – Confine
    E – Extinguish.

Nursing process step: Implementation

Client needs category: Safe, effective care environment

Client needs subcategory: Safety and infection control

Cognitive level: Comprehension

11. The nurse is instructing a client with left-sided weakness on how to use a cane. The nurse should instruct the client to hold the cane on which side?

_____

ANSWER: Right

_____

Rationale: The cane should be held on the stronger side – in this case, the right side – to minimize stress on the affected extremity and to provide a wide base of support.

Nursing process step: Implementation

Client needs category: Physiological integrity

Client needs subcategory: Basic care and comfort

Cognitive level: Application

---

12. A 20-year-old male seeks care at a local emergency care center after spraining his ankle while playing football with his friends. The ankle is painful and swollen. Following the physician's order, the nurse initially applies what kind of thermal therapy to relieve the pain?

_____

ANSWER: Cold

_____

Rationale: Pain caused by an injury is best treated initially with cold applications. Cold reduces localized swelling and decreases vasodilation. Decreasing vasodilation prevents pain-producing chemicals from being carried into the circulation.

Nursing process step: Implementation

Client needs category: Physiological integrity

Client needs subcategory: Basic care and comfort

Cognitive level: Application

Basic psychosocial needs

1. The nurse receives a change-of-shift report for a 76-year-old client who had a total hip replacement. The client is not oriented to time, place, or person and is attempting to get out of bed and pull out an I.V. line that's supplying hydration and antibiotics. The client has a vest restraint and bilateral soft wrist restraints. Which of the following actions by the nurse would be appropriate?

Select all that apply:

☐ **A.** Assess and document the behavior that requires continued use of restraints.

☐ **B.** Tie the restraints in quick-release knots.

☐ **C.** Tie the restraints to the side rails of the bed.

☐ **D.** Ask the client if he needs to go to the bathroom and provide range-of-motion exercises every 2 hours.

☐ **E.** Position the vest restraints so that the straps are crossed in the back.

ANSWER: A, B, D

Rationale: The client must be frequently reassessed to determine whether he is ready to have the restraints removed. The information should also be documented. Restraints should be tied in knots that can be released quickly and easily. Toileting and range-of-motion exercises should be performed every 2 hours while a client is in restraints. Restraints should never be secured to side rails because doing so can cause injury if the side rail is lowered without untying the restraint. A vest restraint should be positioned so the straps cross in front of the client, not in the back.

Nursing process step: Implementation

Client needs category: Safe, effective care environment

Client needs subcategory: Safety and infection control

Cognitive level: Application

---

2. A 62-year-old client has just been diagnosed with terminal cancer and is being transferred to home hospice care. The client's daughter tells the nurse, "I don't know what to say to my mother if she asks me if she's going to die." Which of the following responses by the nurse would be appropriate?

Select all that apply:

☐ **A.** "Don't worry, your mother still has some time left."

☐ **B.** "Let's talk about your mother's illness and how it will progress."

☐ **C.** "You sound like you have some questions about your mother dying. Let's talk about that."

☐ **D.** "Don't worry, hospice will take care of your mother."

☐ **E.** "Tell me how you're feeling about your mother dying."

ANSWER: B, C, E

Rationale: Conveying information and providing clear communication can alleviate fears and strengthen the individual's sense of control. Encouraging verbalization of feelings helps build a therapeutic relationship based on trust and reduces anxiety. Telling the daughter not to worry ignores her feelings and discourages further communication.

Nursing process step: Implementation

Client needs category: Psychosocial integrity

Client needs subcategory: Coping and adaptation

Cognitive level: Analysis

3. While providing care to a 26-year-old married female, the nurse notes multiple ecchymotic areas on her arms and trunk. The color of the ecchymotic areas ranges from blue to purple to yellow. When asked by the nurse how she got these bruises, the client responds, "Oh, I tripped." How should the nurse respond?

Select all that apply:

☐ **A.** Document the client's statement and complete a body map indicating the size, color, shape, location, and type of injuries.

☐ **B.** Report suspicions of abuse to the local authorities.

☐ **C.** Assist the client in developing a safety plan for times of increased violence.

☐ **D.** Call the client's husband to discuss the situation.

☐ **E.** Tell the client that she needs to leave the abusive situation as soon as possible.

☐ **F.** Provide the client with telephone numbers of local shelters and safe houses.

ANSWER: A, C, F

Rationale: The nurse should objectively document her assessment findings. A detailed description of physical findings of abuse in the medical record is essential if legal action is pursued. All women suspected to be victims of abuse should be counseled on a safety plan, which consists of recognizing escalating violence within the family and formulating a plan to exit quickly. The nurse should not report this suspicion of abuse because the client is a competent adult who has the right to self-determination. Nurses do, however, have a duty to report cases of actual or suspected abuse in children or elderly clients. Contacting the client's husband without her consent violates confidentiality. The nurse should respond to the client in a non-threatening manner that promotes trust, rather than ordering her to break off her relationship.

Nursing process step: Implementation

Client needs category: Psychosocial integrity

Client needs subcategory: Psychosocial adaptation

Cognitive level: Analysis

---

4. Elisabeth Kubler-Ross identifies five stages of death and dying. Loss, grief, and intense sadness are symptoms of which stage?

ANSWER: Depression

Rationale: According to Kubler-Ross, the five stages of death and dying are denial and isolation, anger, bargaining, depression, and acceptance. Loss, grief, and intense sadness indicate depression.

Nursing process step: Data collection

Client needs category: Psychosocial integrity

Client needs subcategory: Coping and adaptation

Cognitive level: Application

5. A 26-year-old client with chronic renal failure plans to receive a kidney transplant. Recently, the physician told the client that he is a poor candidate for transplant because of chronic uncontrolled hypertension and diabetes mellitus. Now, the client tells the nurse, "I want to go off dialysis. I'd rather not live than be on this treatment for the rest of my life." Which of the following responses is appropriate?

Select all that apply:

- ☐ **A.** Take a seat next to the client and sit quietly.
- ☐ **B.** Say to the client, "We all have days when we don't feel like going on."
- ☐ **C.** Leave the room to allow the client to collect his thoughts.
- ☐ **D.** Say to the client, "You're feeling upset about the news you got about the transplant."
- ☐ **E.** Say to the client, "The treatments are only 3 days a week. You can live with that."

ANSWER: A, D

Rationale: Silence is a therapeutic communication technique that allows the nurse and client to reflect on what has taken place or been said. By waiting quietly and attentively, the nurse encourages the client to initiate and maintain conversation. By reflecting the client's implied feelings, the nurse promotes communication. Using such platitudes as "We all have days when we don't feel like going on" fails to address the client's needs. The nurse should not leave the client alone because he may harm himself. Reminding the client of the treatment frequency doesn't address his feelings.

Nursing process step: Implementation

Client needs category: Psychosocial integrity

Client needs subcategory: Coping and adaptation

Cognitive level: Analysis

---

6. The nurse is collecting data on a newly admitted client. When filling out the family assessment, who should the nurse consider to be a part of the client's family?

Select all that apply:

- ☐ **A.** People related by blood or marriage
- ☐ **B.** All the people whom the client views as family
- ☐ **C.** People who live in the same house
- ☐ **D.** People who the nurse thinks are important to the client
- ☐ **E.** People who live in the same house with the same racial background as the client
- ☐ **F.** People who provide for the physical and emotional needs of the client

ANSWER: B, F

Rationale: When providing care to a client, the nurse should consider family members to be all the people whom the client views as family. Family members may also include those people who provide for the physical and emotional needs of the client. The traditional definition of a family has changed and may include people not related by blood or marriage, those of a different racial background, and those who may not live in the same house as the client. Family members are defined by the client, not by the nurse.

Nursing process step: Data collection

Client needs category: Health promotion and maintenance

Client needs subcategory: Growth and development through the life span

Cognitive level: Analysis

7. The nurse is caring for a client whose cultural background is different from her own. Which of the following actions are appropriate?

Select all that apply:

☐ **A.** Consider that nonverbal cues, such as eye contact, may have a different meaning in different cultures.

☐ **B.** Respect the client's cultural beliefs.

☐ **C.** Ask the client if he has cultural or religious requirements that should be considered in his care.

☐ **D.** Explain the nurse's beliefs so that the client will understand the differences.

M E. Understand that all cultures experience pain in the same way.

ANSWER: A, B, C

Rationale: Nonverbal cues may have different meanings in different cultures. In one culture, eye contact is a sign of disrespect; in another, eye contact shows respect and attentiveness. The nurse should always respect the client's cultural beliefs and ask if he has cultural requirements. This may include food choices or restrictions, body coverings, or time for prayer. The nurse should attempt to understand the client's culture; it is not the client's responsibility to understand the nurse's culture. The nurse should never impose her own beliefs on her clients. Culture influences a client's experience with pain. For example, in one culture pain may be openly expressed whereas in another culture it may be quietly endured.

Nursing process step: Planning

Client needs category: Psychosocial integrity

Client needs subcategory: Coping and adaptation

Cognitive level: Analysis

---

8. The nurse is caring for a 45-year-old married woman who has undergone hemicolectomy for colon cancer. The woman has two children. Which of the following concepts about families should the nurse keep in mind when providing care for this client?

Select all that apply:

☐ **A.** Illness in one family member can affect all members.

☐ **B.** Family roles don't change because of illness.

☐ **C.** A family member may have more than one role at a time in a family.

☐ **D.** Children typically aren't affected by adult illness.

☐ **E.** The effects of an illness on a family depend on the stage of the family's life cycle.

☐ **F.** Changes in sleeping and eating patterns may be signs of stress in a family.

ANSWER: A, C, E, F

Rationale: Illness in one family member can affect all family members, even children. Each member of a family may have several roles to perform. A middle-aged woman, for example, may have the roles of mother, wage-earner, wife, and housekeeper. Families move through certain predictable life cycles (such as birth of a baby, a growing family, adult children leaving home, and grandparenting). The impact of illness on the family may depend on the stage of the life cycle as family members take on different roles and the family structure changes. Illness produces stress in families; changes in eating and sleeping patterns are signs of stress. When one family member can't fulfill a role due to illness, the roles of the other family members are affected.

Nursing process step: Implementation

Client needs category: Health promotion and maintenance

Client needs subcategory: Growth and development through the life span

Cognitive level: Analysis

9. The nurse is performing a nursing assessment on a 72-year-old client admitted with end-stage renal failure. The nurse asks the client if he has a legal document that provides instructions for his care (living will) and names a durable power of attorney for health care if the client cannot act for himself. What is the name of this document?

_____

ANSWER: Advance directive

Rationale: An advance directive is a legal document that's used as a guideline for life-sustaining medical care of a client with an advanced disease or disability who is no longer able to indicate his own wishes. An advance directive includes the living will, which instructs the physician to administer no life-sustaining treatment, and a durable power of attorney for health care, which names another person to act in the client's behalf for medical decisions in the event that the client can't act for himself.

Nursing process step: Data collection

Client needs category: Safe, effective care environment

Client needs subcategory: Coordinated care

Cognitive level: Comprehension

---

10. A nurse is working with the family of a client who has Alzheimer's disease. The nurse notes that the client's spouse is too exhausted to continue providing care all alone. The adult children live too far away to provide relief on a weekly basis. Which nursing interventions would be most helpful?

Select all that apply:

- ☐ **A.** Calling a family meeting to tell the absent children that they must participate in helping the client

- ☐ **B.** Suggesting the spouse seek psychological counseling to help cope with exhaustion

- ☐ **C.** Recommending community resources for adult day care and respite care

- ☐ **D.** Encouraging the spouse to talk about the difficulties involved in caring for a loved one with Alzheimer's disease

- ☐ **E.** Asking whether friends or church members can help with errands or provide short periods of relief

- ☐ **F.** Recommending that the client be placed in a long-term care facility

ANSWER: C, D, E

Rationale: Many community services exist for Alzheimer's clients and their families. Encouraging use of these resources may make it possible for the client to stay at home and to alleviate the spouse's exhaustion. The nurse can also support the caregiver by urging her to talk about the difficulties she's facing in caring for a spouse. Friends and church members may be able to help provide care to the client, allowing the caregiver time for rest, exercise, or an enjoyable activity. A family meeting to tell the children to participate more would probably be ineffective and may evoke anger or guilt. Counseling may be helpful, but it wouldn't alleviate the caregiver's physical exhaustion and wouldn't address the client's immediate needs. A long-term care facility is not an option until the family is ready to make that decision.

Nursing process step: Implementation

Client needs category: Psychosocial integrity

Client needs subcategory: Coping and adaptation

Cognitive level: Analysis

Medication and I.V. administration

1. A 64-year-old client has just had total hip replacement surgery. The physician orders heparin 8,000 units to be administered subcutaneously. The label on the heparin vial reads: heparin 10,000 units/ml. How many milliliters of heparin should the nurse draw up in the syringe to administer the correct dose?

ANSWER: 0.8

Rationale: The following formula is used to calculate drug dosages:

dose on hand/quantity on hand = dose desired/X

In this example, the equation is as follows:

10,000 units/ml = 8,000 units/X; X = 0.8 ml.

Nursing process step: Implementation

Client needs category: Physiological integrity

Client needs subcategory: Pharmacological therapies

Cognitive level: Application

2. After laparoscopic cholecystectomy, a 43-year-old client complains of pain and nausea. The nurse is preparing meperidine hydrochloride (Demerol) 75 mg and promethazine hydrochloride (Phenergan) 12.5 mg to be administered intramuscularly in the same syringe. If the label on the Demerol reads 50 mg/ml and the label on the Phenergan reads 25 mg/ml, how many milliliters should the nurse have in the syringe after the correct doses are drawn up?

ANSWER: 2

Rationale: The following formula is used to calculate drug dosages:

dose on hand/quantity on hand = dose desired/X

In this example, the formula for calculating the amount of Demerol is as follows:

50 mg/ml = 75 mg/X; X = 1.5 ml.

The formula for calculating the amount of Phenergan is as follows:

25 mg/ml = 12.5 mg/X; X = 0.5 ml.

To calculate the total milliliters that should be drawn up in the syringe, the nurse adds the quantity of Demerol and the quantity of Phenergan, as follows:

1.5 ml + 0.5 ml = 2 ml total drawn up in the syringe.

Nursing process step: Implementation

Client needs category: Physiological integrity

Client needs subcategory: Pharmacological therapies

Cognitive level: Application

3. The nurse gives the client an I.M. injection above and outside an imaginary line drawn from the posterior superior iliac spine to the greater trochanter of the femur. Which I.M. site did the nurse use?

_____

ANSWER: Dorsogluteal

Rationale: The nurse can identify the dorsogluteal I.M. injection site by drawing an imaginary line from the posterior superior iliac spine to the greater trochanter of the femur. The injection is administered above and outside the line.

Nursing process step: Implementation

Client needs category: Physiological integrity

Client needs subcategory: Pharmacological therapies

Cognitive level: Knowledge

---

4. The nurse is administering ampicillin (Polycillin) 125 mg I.M. every 6 hours to a 10-kg child with a respiratory tract infection. The drug label reads, "The recommended dose for a client weighing less than 40 kg is 25 mg to 50 mg/kg/day I.M. or I.V. in equally divided doses at 6- to 8-hour intervals." The drug concentration is 125 mg/5 ml. Which nursing interventions are appropriate at this time?

Select all that apply:

☐ **A.** Draw up 10 ml of ampicillin to administer.

☐ **B.** Administer the medication at 10:00 a.m., 2:00 p.m., 6:00 p.m., and 10:00 p.m.

☐ **C.** Assess the client for allergies to penicillin.

☐ **D.** Administer the medication because it's within the dosing recommendations.

☐ **E.** Question the physician about the order because it's more than the recommended dosage.

☐ **F.** Obtain a sputum culture before administering the medication.

ANSWER: C, D, F

Rationale: Because ampicillin is a penicillin antibiotic, the client should be assessed for allergy to penicillin before the medication is administered. The dose of ampicillin is within the recommended range for a 10-kg client: 50 mg/kg X 10 kg = 500 mg. A dose of 500 mg divided by 4 (given every 6 hours) = 125 mg, which is within the recommended range. Cultures should be obtained before antibiotics are given. The nurse should draw up 5 ml to administer the correct dose, according to the concentration on the label. The dosing schedule in option B is in 4-hour intervals and shouldn't be used because the recommended dosing is in 6- to 8-hour intervals.

Nursing process step: Implementation

Client needs category: Physiological integrity

Client needs subcategory: Pharmacological therapies

Cognitive level: Analysis

5. The nurse is using the Z-track method of I.M. injection to administer iron dextran to a client with iron deficiency anemia. Which of the following techniques should the nurse use to give this injection?

Select all that apply:

☐ **A.** Confirm the client's identity before administering the iron dextran.

☐ **B.** Inject the iron dextran into the deltoid muscle.

☐ **C.** Change the needle after drawing up the iron dextran.

☐ **D.** Before inserting the needle, displace the skin laterally by pulling it away from the injection site.

☐ **E.** Inject the iron dextran after aspirating for a blood return.

☐ **F.** After removing the needle, massage the injection site.

ANSWER: A, C, D, E

Rationale: Before administering any medication, the nurse confirms the client's identity. After drawing up iron dextran, she removes the first needle and attaches a second needle to prevent tracking the medication through the subcutaneous tissue when the needle is inserted. To administer the injection by Z-track method, the nurse first displaces the skin laterally by pulling it away from the injection site. The nurse should aspirate for a blood return before administering iron dextran; if no blood appears, the medication may be injected. Iron dextran should be administered into the large dorsogluteal muscle only. After injecting iron dextran, the nurse shouldn't massage the site because this could force the medication into the subcutaneous tissue.

Nursing process step: Implementation

Client needs category: Physiological integrity

Client needs subcategory: Pharmacological therapies

Cognitive level: Application

---

6. The nurse is preparing to administer regular insulin 4 units to a client with type 1 diabetes mellitus. Which of the following equipment does the nurse need to perform the injection?

Select all that apply:

☐ **A.** Medication administration record

☐ **B.** Nursing assessment sheet

☐ **C.** 27-gauge, ½" needle

☐ **D.** 22-gauge, ½" needle

☐ **E.** 27-gauge, 1" needle

☐ **F.** 22-gauge 1" needle

ANSWER: A AND C

Rationale: To administer medication, the nurse needs the medication administration record to verify the correct client, medication, dose, time, and route. A subcutaneous injection, such as insulin, is administered with a 25-gauge to 27-gauge, ⅝" to ½" needle. The nursing assessment sheet isn't necessary for administering insulin. A 22-gauge needle is too large for a subcutaneous injection. A 1" needle will deliver the medication into muscle rather than subcutaneous tissue.

Nursing process step: Implementation

Client needs category: Physiological integrity

Client needs subcategory: Pharmacological therapies

Cognitive level: Application

7. The nurse is administering insulin to a client with type 1 diabetes mellitus. Identify the tissue layer where placement of the tip of the needle should be to deliver this medication to the proper tissue.

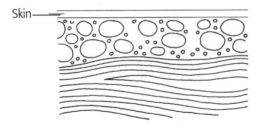

ANSWER:

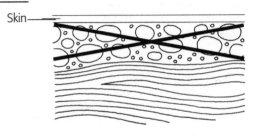

Rationale: Insulin is administered by subcutaneous injection. The tip of the needle should be in the subcutaneous tissue.

Nursing process step: Implementation

Client needs category: Physiological integrity

Client needs subcategory: Pharmacological therapies

Cognitive level: Comprehension

---

8. After cardiac catheterization, a client is to receive 1 L of normal saline solution over 6 hours. If the drop factor for the tubing is 10 drops/ml, how many drops/minute should the nurse set the I.V. infusion for?

ANSWER: 28

Rationale: The following equation is used:

$$\text{drip rate in drops/minute} = \text{ml of solution/minutes} \times \text{drops per/ml}$$

In this case, the formula should read:

$$1{,}000 \text{ ml/360 minutes} \times 10 \text{ drops/ml/hour} = 27.78 \text{ (or 28 drops per minute)}$$

Nursing process step: Implementation

Client needs category: Physiological integrity

Client needs subcategory: Pharmacological therapies

Cognitive level: Application

9. A client with an I.V. line in place complains of pain at the insertion site. Assessment of the site reveals a vein that is red, warm, and hard. Which of the following actions should the nurse take?

Select all that apply:

☐ **A.** Slow the infusion rate.

☐ **B.** Discontinue the infusion.

☐ **C.** Restart the infusion distal to the discontinued I.V. site.

☐ **D.** Restart the infusion in the opposite arm.

☐ **E.** Apply warm soaks to the I.V. site.

☐ **F.** Document assessment of the I.V. site, the nurse's actions, and the client's response to the situation.

ANSWER: B, D, E, F

Rationale: Redness, warmth, pain, and a hard, cord-like vein at the I.V. insertion site suggest that the client has phlebitis. The nurse should discontinue the I.V. line and insert a new I.V. catheter proximal to or above the discontinued I.V. site or in the other arm. Applying warm soaks to the site reduces inflammation. The nurse should document assessment of the I.V. site, actions taken, and the client's response to the situation. When phlebitis is present, slowing the infusion rate won't reduce the phlebitis. Restarting the infusion at a site distal to the phlebitis may contribute to the inflammation.

Nursing process step: Implementation

Client needs category: Physiological integrity

Client needs subcategory: Pharmacological therapies

Cognitive level: Application

---

10. The nurse is administering an I.M. injection into the vastus lateralis muscle. Identify the area where the nurse will inject the medication.

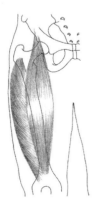

ANSWER:

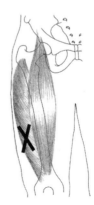

Rationale: The vastus lateralis is an I.M. injection site located in the middle third of the outer aspect of the thigh, from a handbreadth below the greater trochanter to a handbreadth above the knee.

Nursing process step: Implementation

Client needs category: Physiological integrity

Client needs subcategory: Pharmacological therapies

Cognitive level: Application

11. An elderly client comes to the clinic asking for a flu shot. After the physician orders the medication, the nurse prepares the injection and plans to administer it into the client's arm. Which muscle is most appropriate for the nurse to use?

_____

Answer: Deltoid

Rationale: The deltoid muscle is used most frequently for immunizations such as flu shots. It's located on the lateral aspect of the upper arm, 1″ to 2″ below the acromion process of the shoulder.

Nursing process step: Planning

Client needs category: Physiological integrity

Client needs subcategory: Pharmacological therapies

Cognitive level: Application

---

12. When administering an injection into the deltoid muscle, the nurse knows that the maximum amount of milliliters of medication that can be administered into the deltoid muscle is what?

_____

Answer: 2

Rationale: The deltoid muscle is usually the site for injecting a small amount of medication. If more than 2 ml is given in the deltoid muscle, there is a risk of brachial artery and nerve damage.

Nursing process step: Implementation

Client needs category: Physiological integrity

Client needs subcategory: Reduction of risk potential

Cognitive level: Knowledge

13. The nurse transcribes the following physician's order onto the client's medication record:

> March 15, 2003
> Administer 10 gtt of timolol maleate (Timoptic) ophthalmic solution AU daily.
> John Bloom, MD

Which components of the medication order should the nurse question?

Select all that apply:

☐ **A.** Number of drops

☐ **B.** Route

☐ **C.** Type of medication

☐ **D.** Signature

☐ **E.** Frequency of administration

☐ **F.** Date

ANSWER: A, B

Rationale: To ensure that medication errors don't occur, it's important for the nurse to follow the six rights to safe medication administration: right drug, right dose, right route, right time, right client, and right documentation. The number of drops is too great to be instilled into the eye. The medication wouldn't be effective because the dose is too large and would run out. Normally, the physician orders 1 or 2 drops to be instilled into the eye. The correct abbreviation for both eyes is OU. As the order is written, the eye medication would be administered in both ears (AU).

Nursing process step: Evaluation

Client needs category: Safe, effective care environment

Client needs subcategory: Safety and infection control

Cognitive level: Analysis

Basic physical assessment

1. An adolescent client seeks medical attention because of a sore throat and probable mononucleosis. The nurse palpates the client's submandibular lymph nodes for enlargement. Identify the area where the nurse should palpate to best feel these nodes.

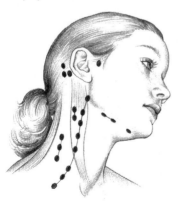

ANSWER:

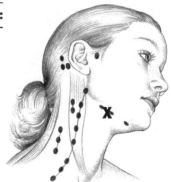

Rationale: The submandibular lymph nodes are located beneath the mandible, or lower jaw, halfway to the chin. These nodes may be enlarged in a client with a throat infection or mononucleosis.

Nursing process step: Data collection

Client needs category: Physiological integrity

Client needs subcategory: Physiological adaptation

Cognitive level: Knowledge

2. A 60-year-old client comes to the clinic seeking medical attention for a rash. The nurse assesses the rash and finds that the client's back and right side are covered with elevated, round, blisterlike lesions that are filled with clear fluid. What medical term should the nurse use to describe these lesions?

_____

ANSWER: Vesicles

Rationale: Vesicles are described as raised, round, serous-filled lesions that are usually no larger than 1 cm in diameter. Examples of vesicles include chickenpox (varicella) and shingles (herpes zoster).

Nursing process step: Data collection

Client needs category: Health promotion and maintenance

Client needs subcategory: Prevention and early detection of disease

Cognitive level: Comprehension

---

3. An elderly client is admitted to the hospital for a fractured hip. He has a history of aortic stenosis. Identify the area where the nurse should place the stethoscope to best hear the murmur.

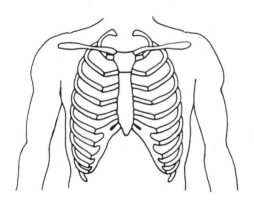

ANSWER:

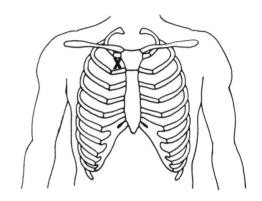

Rationale: The murmur of aortic stenosis is low-pitched, rough, and rasping. It's loudest in the second intercostal space, to the right of the sternum.

Nursing process step: Data collection

Client needs category: Health promotion and maintenance

Client needs subcategory: Prevention and early detection of disease

Cognitive level: Application

4. The nurse is collecting data on a client who has a rash on his chest and upper arms. Which questions should the nurse ask in order to obtain more information about the client's rash?

Select all that apply:

☐ **A.** "When did the rash start?"

☐ **B.** "Are you allergic to any medications, foods, or pollen?"

☐ **C.** "How old are you?"

☐ **D**. "What have you been using to treat the rash?"

☐ **E.** "Have you traveled outside of the country?"

☐ **F.** "Do you smoke cigarettes or drink alcohol?"

ANSWER: A, B, D, E

Rationale: Finding out when the rash first appeared helps the physician make a diagnosis and determine at what stage in the disease process the rash is. Obtaining an allergy history is necessary because rashes related to allergies can occur when a client changes medications, eats new foods, or has contact with allergens in the air (such as pollen). How the client has been treating the rash is important because topical ointments and oral medications may make the rash worse. Travel outside of the country exposes the client to foreign foods and environments that can contribute to the onset of a rash. The client's age and smoking or drinking habits have no real value in determining the cause of the rash.

Nursing process step: Data collection

Client needs category: Physiological integrity

Client needs subcategory: Physiological adaptation

Cognitive level: Application

---

5. An elderly client comes to the clinic complaining of hearing loss. The nurse performs Weber's test to assess the client's ability to hear. Identify the location where the nurse should place the tuning fork to perform this test.

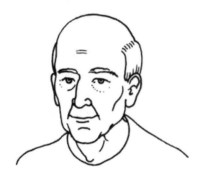

ANSWER:

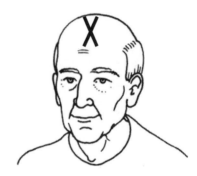

Rationale: To perform Weber's test, the tuning fork should be struck and then placed on the midline of the head. Weber's test determines if sound is heard equally in both ears. If the client hears the sound louder in one ear, he probably has unequal hearing loss that requires further intervention.

Nursing process step: Implementation

Client needs category: Health promotion and maintenance

Client needs subcategory: Prevention and early detection of disease

Cognitive level: Knowledge

6. An 80-year-old client comes to the clinic complaining of shortness of breath. When listening to the client's lungs, the nurse hears intermittent, high- and low-pitched popping sounds in the lower bases of the lungs during inspiration. What term should the nurse use to document these findings?

_____

ANSWER: Crackles

Rationale: Crackles are typically heard on inspiration, can be low- or high-pitched, and occur when air is drawn through fluid in the lung's passageways. They can be classified as fine or course.

Nursing process step: Data collection

Client needs category: Physiological integrity

Client needs subcategory: Physiological adaptation

Cognitive level: Application

---

7. A 40-year-old client is admitted with a diagnosis of new-onset atrial fibrillation. To obtain an accurate pulse count, the nurse counts the apical heart rate. Identify the area where the nurse should place the stethoscope to best hear the apical rate.

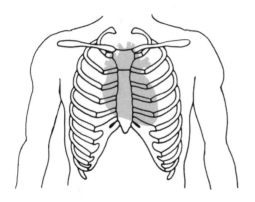

ANSWER:

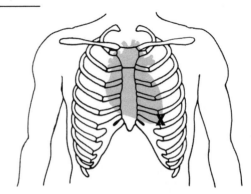

Rationale: The apical heart rate is best heard at the point of maximal impulse, which is generally in the fifth intercostal space at the midclavicular line.

Nursing process step: Data collection

Client needs category: Health promotion and maintenance

Client needs subcategory: Prevention and early detection of disease

Cognitive level: Application

8. An elderly client who is 5'4" and weighs 145 lb is admitted to the long-term care facility. The admitting nurse takes this report: The client sits for long periods in his wheelchair and has bowel and bladder incontinence. He is able to feed himself and has a fair appetite, eating best at breakfast and poorly thereafter. He doesn't have family members living nearby and is often noted to be crying and depressed. He also frequently requires large doses of sedatives.

Which factors place the client at risk for developing a pressure ulcer?

Select all that apply:

☐ **A.** Weight

☐ **B.** Incontinence

☐ **C.** Sitting for long periods of time

☐ **D.** Sedation

☐ **E.** Crying and depression

☐ **F.** Eating poorly at lunch and dinner

Rationale: Inactivity, immobility, incontinence, and sedation are all risk factors for developing pressure ulcers. The client's weight and poor eating habits at lunch and dinner aren't directly related to the risk of developing pressure ulcers, but a calorie count should be taken to see if the client is getting adequate calories and fluids because poor nutrition can contribute to pressure ulcers. The fact that the client cries and is depressed has no direct bearing on this client's risk for developing a pressure ulcer. However, clients with depression are commonly not as active, so his activity levels should be monitored closely.

Nursing process step: Data collection

Client needs category: Physiological integrity

Client needs subcategory: Reduction of risk potential

Cognitive level: Analysis

---

9. The nurse finds a client lying on the floor of the hospital corridor. After determining unconsciousness, breathlessness, and providing two ventilations, the nurse checks the client's carotid artery for a pulse. Identify the area where the nurse can best palpate the carotid pulse.

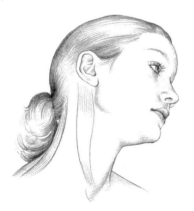

ANSWER:

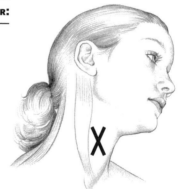

Rationale: The carotid artery is located in the neck in the groove between the trachea and the sternocleidomastoid muscle. It's the artery of choice for determining a pulse in this situation because it's usually the most accessible.

Nursing process step: Data collection

Client needs category: Physiological integrity

Client needs subcategory: Physiological adaptation

Cognitive level: Knowledge

10. A diabetic client comes to the clinic for medical attention because of numbness and tingling in his lower extremities. The nurse obtains the client's vital signs and palpates the dorsalis pedis pulse. Identify the area where the nurse places her fingers to palpate the pedal pulse.

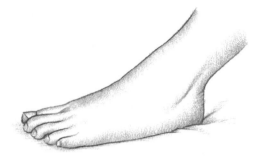

ANSWER:

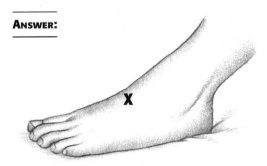

Rationale: The pedal pulse is located on the top portion of the foot. Because clients with diabetes have complications related to circulation in the lower extremities, health care providers should palpate pedal pulses and check capillary refill.

Nursing process step: Data collection

Client needs category: Health promotion and maintenance

Client needs subcategory: Prevention and early detection of disease

Cognitive level: Knowledge

---

11. An adolescent boy comes to the emergency department seeking medical attention for severe pain located in the area of the appendix. Identify the area where the nurse would expect the pain to localize.

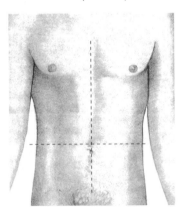

ANSWER:

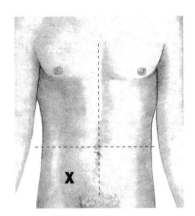

Rationale: Pain and tenderness during an acute attack of appendicitis localize in the right lower quadrant, midway between the umbilicus and the crest of the ilium.

Nursing process step: Implementation

Client needs category: Physiological integrity

Client needs subcategory: Physiological adaptation

Cognitive level: Knowledge

12. A 35-year-old client is admitted to the hospital for routine outpatient surgery. Before surgery, the nurse auscultates the client's chest for breath sounds. Identify the area where the nurse should expect to hear bronchovesicular breath sounds.

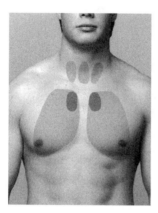

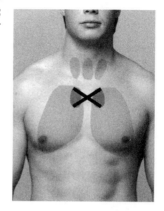

Rationale: Bronchovesicular breath sounds are best heard next to the upper third of the sternum and between the scapulae. These breath sounds are equal in length during inspiration and expiration.

Nursing process step: Data collection

Client needs category: Health promotion and maintenance

Client needs subcategory: Prevention and early detection of disease

Cognitive level: Knowledge

Part 2
Medical-surgical nursing

1. A 52-year-old client with a history of hypertension has just had a total hip replacement. The physician orders hydrochlorothiazide (Hydro-Chlor) 35 mg oral solution by mouth, once a day. The label on the solution reads hydrochlorothiazide 50 mg/5 ml. To administer the correct dose, how many ml should the nurse pour?

_____

ANSWER: 3.5

Rationale: The correct formula to calculate a drug dosage is:

dose on hand/quantity on hand = dose desired/X.

In this example, the equation is:

50 mg/5 ml = 35 mg/X; X = 3.5 ml.

Nursing process step: Implementation

Client needs category: Physiological integrity

Client needs subcategory: Pharmacological therapies

Cognitive level: Application

2. A client is prescribed furosemide (Lasix) to manage his heart failure. The nurse notes that the client has not been receiving any supplemental electrolytes. What laboratory value should the nurse check before administering this medication?

_____

ANSWER: Potassium

Rationale: Because loop diuretics, such as furosemide, promote excretion of potassium, the nurse should monitor serum potassium levels. Potassium replacement therapy may be necessary to prevent hypokalemia.

Nursing process step: Data collection

Client needs category: Physiological integrity

Client needs subcategory: Pharmacological therapies

Cognitive level: Comprehension

3. The nurse is assessing a client who is at risk for cardiac tamponade due to chest trauma sustained in a motorcycle accident. What is the client's pulse pressure if his blood pressure is 108/82 mm Hg?

_____

ANSWER: 26

Rationale: Pulse pressure is the difference between systolic and diastolic pressures. Normally, systolic pressure exceeds diastolic pressure by about 40 mm Hg. Narrowed pulse pressure, a difference of less than 30 mm Hg, is a sign of cardiac tamponade.

Nursing process step: Data collection

Client needs category: Physiological integrity

Client needs subcategory: Physiological adaptation

Cognitive level: Application

---

4. The nurse is assessing a client with heart failure. Which heart valve sound will the nurse hear best at the fifth left intercostal space at the midclavicular line?

_____

ANSWER: Mitral

Rationale: Closure of the mitral valve (along with closure of the tricuspid valve) produces the first heart sound, which is called S_1. It's best heard on the left side of the chest, at the fifth intercostal space at the midclavicular line.

Nursing process step: Data collection

Client needs category: Physiological integrity

Client needs subcategory: Physiological adaptation

Cognitive level: Comprehension

5. A client is assisting with receiving heparin I.V. for the treatment of thrombophlebitis. Which laboratory value should the nurse monitor to evaluate the drug's effectiveness?

_____

ANSWER: Partial thromboplastin time

Rationale: Heparin is at a therapeutic level when partial thromboplastin time is 1 ½ to 2 times the control.

Nursing process step: Data collection

Client needs category: Physiological integrity

Client needs subcategory: Pharmacological therapies

Cognitive level: Comprehension

---

6. The nurse is caring for a client who just underwent cardiac catheterization through a femoral access site. Which nursing interventions should the nurse include in the care plan for the next 8 hours?

Select all that apply:

☐ **A.** Maintain pressure over the femoral access site.

☑ **B.** Allow the client to sit upright for meals.

☑ **C.** Check the dressing and access site for bleeding.

☐ **D.** Monitor vital signs every 4 hours.

☑ **E.** Keep the extremity straight.

☐ **F.** Allow use of the bedside commode.

ANSWER: A, C, E

Rationale: Pressure should be applied at the access site to control bleeding and promote clot formation. The dressing and access site must be observed frequently for bleeding and hematoma formation. When the femoral access site is used, the head of the bed may not be raised greater than 30 degrees and the affected leg must be kept extended. Therefore, the client may not sit upright for meals or use the bedside commode. Following this procedure, the nurse should monitor vital signs every 15 minutes for the first hour, every 30 minutes for the next 2 hours, and every 4 hours after that.

Nursing process step: Planning

Client needs category: Physiological integrity

Client needs subcategory: Reduction of risk potential

Cognitive level: Application

7. The nurse is assisting with preparing a teaching plan for a client who recently underwent surgery for insertion of a permanent pacemaker. Which of the following instructions should the nurse include in the teaching plan?

Select all that apply:

☑ **A.** Check heart rate for 1 minute daily.

☐ **B.** Check respiratory rate for 1 minute daily.

☑ **C.** Report any bulging at the insertion site.

☑ **D.** Report redness, swelling, or discharge at insertion site.

☐ **E.** Stay away from airport metal detectors.

☑ **F.** Avoid magnetic resonance imaging (MRI) diagnostic studies.

ANSWER: A, D, F

Rationale: The client with an implanted pacemaker should assess his heart rate daily and report rates that are too fast or too slow. The nurse should instruct him to inspect the insertion site and report signs and symptoms of infection, such as redness, swelling, and discharge. MRI studies are contraindicated in the client with a permanent pacemaker because the magnet may move the metal pacemaker within the body, causing injury. It isn't necessary to obtain a respiratory rate to assess functioning of a pacemaker. A slight bulge at the pacemaker insertion is normal. It's safe for a client with a pacemaker to go through an airport metal detector, but the pacemaker may activate the metal detector. The client should carry his pacemaker identification card to show to security personnel.

Nursing process step: Planning

Client needs category: Physiological integrity

Client needs subcategory: Reduction of risk potential

Cognitive level: Application

---

8. The nurse is admitting a client with substernal chest pain. Which of the following diagnostic tests does the nurse anticipate the client will receive to confirm or rule out a diagnosis of myocardial infarction (MI)?

Select all that apply:

☐ **A.** Serum bilirubin

☑ **B.** Serum troponin

☑ **C.** Serum myoglobin

☐ **D.** Urinalysis

☐ **E.** Electroencephalogram

☐ **F.** 24-hour creatinine clearance

ANSWER: B AND C

Rationale: Troponin and myoglobin are enzymes that are released when cardiac muscle is damaged. Serum troponin levels increase within 2 to 4 hours after MI. Serum myoglobin levels increase within ½ hour to 2 hours after MI. Serum bilirubin evaluates liver function and is not altered with cardiac damage. Urinalysis and 24-hour creatinine clearance reflect kidney — not cardiac — function. An electroencephalogram evaluates the electrical activity of the brain.

Nursing process step: Data collection

Client needs category: Physiological integrity

Client needs subcategory: Physiological adaptation

Cognitive level: Application

9. Which of the following signs and symptoms should the nurse expect to find in a client with angina?

Select all that apply:

☑ **A.** Chest tightness

☐ **B.** General muscle aching

☐ **C.** Chest pressure

☐ **D.** Jaw pain

☐ **E.** Slowed respiratory rate

☐ **F.** Bradycardia

ANSWER: A, C, D

Rationale: Chest tightness, chest pressure, and jaw pain are all symptoms of angina. General muscle aching is not associated with angina. Respirations and heart rate typically increase, not decrease, with anginal attacks.

Nursing process step: Data collection

Client needs category: Physiological integrity

Client needs subcategory: Physiological adaptation

Cognitive level: Application

---

10. A client is diagnosed with myocardial infarction. Which of the following assessment data indicate that the client has developed left-sided heart failure?

Select all that apply:

☐ **A.** Ascites

☑ **B.** Jugular vein distention

☐ **C.** Orthopnea

☐ **D.** Cough

☐ **E.** Hepatomegaly

☑ **F.** Crackles

ANSWER: C, D, F

Rationale: Left-sided heart failure produces primarily pulmonary signs and symptoms, such as orthopnea, cough, and crackles. Right-sided heart failure primarily produces systemic signs and symptoms, such as ascites, jugular vein distention, and hepatomegaly.

Nursing process step: Data collection

Client needs category: Physiological integrity

Client needs subcategory: Physiological adaptation

Cognitive level: Application

11. The nurse is performing a cardiac assessment on a client with hypertension. Identify the area where the nurse should place the stethoscope to best auscultate the pulmonic valve.

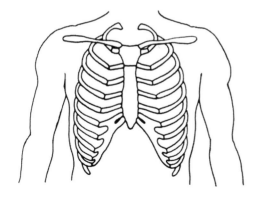

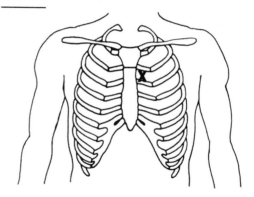

Rationale: Typically, the pulmonic valve is best heard at the second intercostal space, at the left sternal border.

Nursing process step: Data collection

Client needs category: Physiological integrity

Client needs subcategory: Physiological adaptation

Cognitive level: Application

---

12. The nurse is assessing the peripheral pulses of a client who underwent cardiac catheterization through the left groin. Identify the area where the nurse should palpate the left posterior tibial artery.

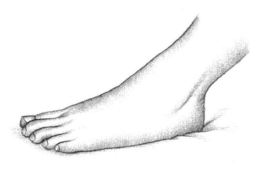

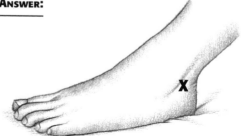

Rationale: The posterior tibial pulse is located behind and just below the lateral malleolus of the foot.

Nursing process step: Data collection

Client needs category: Physiological integrity

Client needs subcategory: Reduction of risk potential

Cognitive level: Application

13. A client with atrial fibrillation is diagnosed with an embolic stroke. Identify the heart chamber that is the most likely source of the fragmented clot responsible for the stroke.

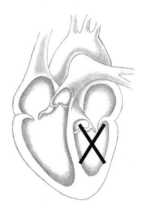

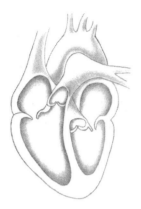

Rationale: Clients with atrial fibrillation are at increased risk for clot formation in the left ventricle of the heart due to stagnation of blood. If a piece of the clot breaks loose and travels to the brain, the client suffers an embolic stroke.

Nursing process step: Data collection

Client needs category: Physiological integrity

Client needs subcategory: Physiological adaptation

Cognitive level: Application

Oncologic disorders

1. A client in the terminal stage of cancer is being transferred to hospice care. Which information should the nurse include in the teaching plan regarding hospice care?

☐ **A.** Care focuses on controlling symptoms and relieving pain.

☐ **B.** A multidisciplinary team provides care.

☐ **C.** Services are provided based on the client's ability to pay.

☐ **D.** Hospice care is provided only in hospice centers.

☐ **E.** Bereavement care is provided to the family.

☐ **F.** Care is provided in the home independent of physicians.

ANSWER: A, B, E

Rationale: Hospice care focuses on controlling symptoms and relieving pain at the end of life. Care is provided by a multidisciplinary team that may consist of nurses, physicians, chaplains, aides, and volunteers. After the client's death, hospice provides bereavement care to the grieving family. Hospice care is provided based on need, not on ability to pay. It's provided in various settings, including hospice centers, homes, hospitals, and long-term care facilities. Care is provided under the direction of a physician, who is a key member of the hospice care team.

Nursing process step: Planning

Client needs category: Physiological integrity

Client needs subcategory: Basic care and comfort

Cognitive level: Application

2. After a client receives chemotherapy for lung cancer, his platelet count falls to 98,000/μl. What term should the nurse use to refer to this drop in the platelet count?

_____

ANSWER: Thrombocytopenia

Rationale: A normal platelet count in adults is 140,000 to 400,000/μl. Chemotherapeutic drugs produce bone marrow depression, resulting in reduced red blood cell counts (anemia), white blood cell counts (leucopenia), and platelet counts (thrombocytopenia).

Nursing process step: Implementation

Client needs category: Physiological integrity

Client needs subcategory: Physiological adaptation

Cognitive level: Comprehension

---

3. After undergoing chemotherapy to treat breast cancer, a client has a white blood cell (WBC) count of 1,300/μl. This client should be placed in which type of isolation?

_____

ANSWER: Reverse

Rationale: The client with a WBC count below 1,500/μl should be placed in reverse isolation to reduce the risk of infection.

Nursing process step: Planning

Client needs category: Safe, effective care environment

Client needs subcategory: Safety and infection control

Cognitive level: Application

4. After having a lobectomy for lung cancer, a client receives a chest tube connected to a three-chamber chest drainage system. The nurse observes that the drainage system is functioning correctly when she notes fluctuations in which compartment of the system when the client breathes?

_____

ANSWER: Water-seal

Rationale: Fluctuations in the water-seal compartment (or tidal movements) indicate normal function of the system as the pressure in the tubing changes with the client's respirations.

Nursing process step: Data collection

Client needs category: Physiological integrity

Client needs subcategory: Reduction of risk potential

Cognitive level: Application

---

5. A client with laryngeal cancer has undergone laryngectomy and is receiving radiation therapy to the head and neck. The nurse should monitor the client for which adverse effects of external radiation?

Select all that apply:

☐ **A.** Xerostomia

☐ **B.** Stomatitis

☐ **C.** Thrombocytopenia

☐ **D.** Cystitis

☐ **E.** Dysgeusia

☐ **F.** Leukopenia

ANSWER: A, B, E

Rationale: Radiation of the head and neck commonly causes xerostomia (dry mouth), stomatitis (irritation of the oral mucous membranes), and dysgeusia (a diminished sense of taste). Thrombocytopenia (reduced platelet count) and leukopenia (reduced white blood cell count) may occur after systemic radiation. Cystitis may occur after radiation of the genitourinary system.

Nursing process step: Data collection

Client needs category: Physiological integrity

Client needs subcategory: Reduction of risk potential

Cognitive level: Application

6. A client with bladder cancer undergoes surgical removal of the bladder and construction of an ileal conduit. Which assessment findings indicate that the client is developing complications?

Select all that apply:

☐ **A.** Urine output is greater than 30 ml/hr.

☑ **B.** The stoma appears dusky.

☐ **C.** The stoma protrudes from the skin.

☐ **D.** Mucus shreds are in the urine collection bag.

☐ **E.** Edema of the stoma is present during the first 24 hours postoperatively.

☑ **F.** The client experiences sharp abdominal pain and rigidity.

ANSWER: B, C, F

Rationale: A dusky appearance of the stoma indicates decreased blood supply; a healthy stoma should appear beefy-red. Protrusion indicates prolapse of the stoma. Sharp abdominal pain and rigidity suggests peritonitis. A urine output greater than 30 ml/hr is a sign of adequate renal perfusion and is a normal finding. Stomal edema is a normal finding during the first 24 hours after surgery. Because mucous membranes are used to create the conduit, mucus in the urine is expected.

Nursing process step: Data collection

Client needs category: Physiological integrity

Client needs subcategory: Reduction of risk potential

Cognitive level: Analysis

---

7. A client receiving chemotherapy for breast cancer develops myelosuppression. Which instructions should the nurse include in the discharge teaching plan?

Select all that apply:

☐ **A.** Avoid people who have recently received attenuated vaccines.

☐ **B.** Avoid activities that may cause bleeding.

☐ **C.** Wash hands frequently.

☐ **D.** Increase intake of fresh fruits and vegetables.

☐ **E.** Avoid crowded places, such as shopping malls.

☐ **F.** Treat a sore throat with over-the-counter products.

ANSWER: A, B, C, E

Rationale: Chemotherapy can cause myelosuppression (reduced numbers of red blood cells, white blood cells, and platelets). Clients receiving chemotherapy need to avoid people who have recently been vaccinated because such interaction may exaggerate myelosuppression. Frequent hand-washing is the best way to prevent the spread of infection. In addition, chemotherapy clients should avoid activities that could cause trauma and bleeding because of their reduced platelet counts. They should also avoid crowded places and people with colds during the flu season because of their reduced ability to fight infection. Fresh fruits and vegetables should be avoided because they can harbor bacteria that aren't easily removed by washing. Signs and symptoms of infection such as a sore throat, fever, or cough should be reported immediately to the physician.

Nursing process step: Planning

Client needs category: Physiological integrity

Client needs subcategory: Reduction of risk potential

Cognitive level: Application

8. What diagnostic study is recommended to be performed annually on all women older than age 50?

_____

Gastrointestinal disorders

1. An 86-year-old client with a history of atrial fibrillation takes 5 mg of warfarin (Coumadin) daily. She comes to the emergency department with a 3-day history of passing black, tarry stools. What term does the triage nurse use to document her stools?

_____

ANSWER: Melena

Rationale: Melena is the term used to describe black, tarry stools.

Nursing process step: Data collection

Client needs category: Physiological integrity

Client needs subcategory: Physiological adaptation

Cognitive level: Knowledge

2. A client comes to the emergency department complaining of transient epigastric pain that radiates to his back and right shoulder. He also experiences burning in his chest after eating fried foods. These symptoms suggest that the client is most likely experiencing what GI disorder?

_____

ANSWER: Cholecystitis

Rationale: Cholecystitis (inflammation of the gallbladder) is characterized by epigastric pain that radiates to the back and right shoulder. This pain commonly occurs after eating foods high in fat, especially those that are fried. A client with cholecystitis may also experience nausea, vomiting, and flatulence.

Nursing process step: Data collection

Client needs category: Physiological integrity

Client needs subcategory: Reduction of risk potential

Cognitive level: Analysis

---

3. As part of a routine screening for colorectal cancer, a client must undergo fecal occult blood testing. Which foods should the nurse instruct the client to avoid 48 to 72 hours before the test and throughout the collection period?

Select all that apply:

☑ **A.** High-fiber foods

☐ **B.** Red meat

☐ **C.** Turnips

☐ **D.** Horseradish

☐ **E.** Tomatoes

☐ **F.** Apples

ANSWER: B, C, D

Rationale: The client should be instructed to maintain a high-fiber diet and to refrain from eating red meat, poultry, fish, turnips, and horseradish for 48 to 72 hours before the test and throughout the collection period.

Nursing process step: Implementation

Client needs category: Health promotion and maintenance

Client needs subcategory: Prevention and early detection of disease

Cognitive level: Application

4. A 58-year-old client with osteoarthritis is admitted to the hospital with peptic ulcer disease. Which findings are commonly associated with peptic ulcer disease?

Select all that apply:

☐ **A.** Localized, colicky periumbilical pain

☐ **B.** History of nonsteroidal anti-inflammatory use

☑ **C.** Epigastric pain that's relieved by antacids

☐ **D.** Tachycardia

☑ **E.** Nausea and weight loss

☐ **F.** Low-grade fever

ANSWER: B, C, E

Rationale: Peptic ulcer disease is characterized by nausea, hematemesis, melena, weight loss, and left-sided epigastric pain—occurring 1 to 2 hours after eating—that's relieved with antacids. Nonsteroidal anti-inflammatory drug use is also associated with peptic ulcer disease. Appendicitis begins with generalized or localized colicky periumbilical or epigastric pain, followed by anorexia, nausea, a few episodes of vomiting, low-grade fever, and tachycardia.

Nursing process step: Data collection

Client needs category: Physiological integrity

Client needs subcategory: Physiological adaptation

Cognitive level: Analysis

---

5. A client undergoes a barium swallow fluoroscopy that confirms gastroesophageal reflux disease (GERD). Based on this diagnosis, the client should be instructed to take which action?

Select all that apply:

☐ **A.** Follow a high-fat, low-fiber diet.

☑ **B.** Avoid caffeine and carbonated beverages.

☐ **C.** Sleep with the head of the bed flat.

☑ **D.** Stop smoking.

☑ **E.** Take antacids 1 hour and 3 hours after meals.

☐ **F.** Limit alcohol consumption to one drink per day.

ANSWER: B, D, E

Rationale: The nurse should instruct the client with GERD to follow a low-fat, high-fiber diet. Caffeine, carbonated beverages, alcohol, and smoking should be avoided because they aggravate GERD. In addition, the client should take antacids as prescribed (typically 1 hour and 3 hours after meals and at bedtime). Lying down with the head of the bed elevated, not flat, reduces intra-abdominal pressure, thereby reducing the symptoms of GERD.

Nursing process step: Implementation

Client needs category: Health promotion and maintenance

Client needs subcategory: Prevention and early detection of disease

Cognitive level: Application

6. A client with constipation is prescribed an irrigating enema. Which steps should the nurse take when administering an enema?

Select all that apply:

☑ **A.** Assist the client into the left-lateral Sims' position.

☑ **B.** Lubricate the distal end of the rectal catheter.

☐ **C.** Warm the solution to 110° F (43.3° C).

☐ **D.** Insert the tube 1" to 1½".

☐ **E.** Administer 250 to 500 ml of irrigating solution.

☑ **F.** Be sure to keep the solution container below 18" above bed level.

ANSWER: A, B, F

Rationale: To administer an enema, the nurse should prepare the prescribed type and amount of solution. The standard volume of an irrigating enema for an adult is 750 to 1,000 ml. For an adult, the solution should be warmed to 100° (37.8° C) to 105° F (40.6° C) to help reduce client discomfort. The nurse should help the client into left-lateral Sims' position. After lubricating the distal end of the rectal catheter, the nurse should insert the tube 2" to 3". During infusion, the solution bag shouldn't be raised higher than 18" above bed level.

Nursing process step: Implementation

Client needs category: Physiological integrity

Client needs subcategory: Basic care and comfort

Cognitive level: Application

---

7. A client with cirrhosis is ordered to have a daily measurement of his abdominal girth. Identify the anatomical landmark where the tape measure should be placed when obtaining this measurement.

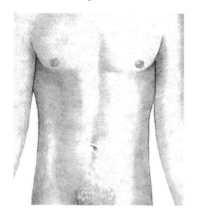

ANSWER:

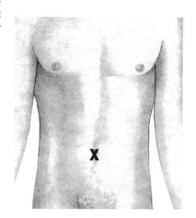

Rationale: Abdominal girth should be measured at the umbilicus to obtain the most accurate measurement. Using any other anatomical landmark wouldn't provide the correct measurement for the client's abdominal girth.

Nursing process step: Data collection

Client needs category: Health promotion and maintenance

Client needs subcategory: Prevention and early detection of disease

Cognitive level: Application

8. A 53-year-old client undergoes colonoscopy for colorectal cancer screening. A polyp was removed during the procedure. Which nursing interventions are necessary when caring for the client immediately after colonoscopy?

Select all that apply:

☐ **A.** When the client recovers from sedation, tell him he must follow a clear liquid diet.

☐ **B.** Instruct the client that he shouldn't drive for 24 hours.

☑ **C.** Observe the client closely for signs and symptoms of bowel perforation.

☑ **D.** Monitor vital signs frequently until they're stable.

☑ **E.** Inform the client that there may be blood in his stool and that he should report excessive blood immediately.

☐ **F.** Tell the client to report excessive flatus.

Answer: C, D, E

Rationale: After colonoscopy, the nurse should observe the client closely for signs and symptoms of bowel perforation (malaise, rectal bleeding, abdominal pain and distention, fever, and mucopurulent drainage). The nurse should monitor vital signs frequently, until they become stable. Because a polyp was removed during the procedure, the nurse should inform the client that there may be some blood in his stool and that he should report excessive bleeding immediately. The nurse should tell the client he might pass large amounts of flatus resulting from air insufflated to distend the colon but it is not necessary to report it. When the client has recovered from sedation, he may resume his usual diet; a clear liquid diet isn't necessary. The client shouldn't drive for 12 hours after being sedated.

Nursing process step: Implementation

Client needs category: Health promotion and maintenance

Client needs subcategory: Prevention and early detection of disease

Cognitive level: Application

---

9. A client's stool specimen is positive for *Clostridium difficile*. Based on this diagnosis, the nurse should observe what type of precautions to prevent the spread of infection?

_____

Answer: Contact

Rationale: *Clostridium difficile* is an infection that's easily transmitted through direct contact or through contact with items in the client's environment. To prevent the spread of infection, clients should be cared for using contact precautions in addition to standard precautions.

Nursing process step: Implementation

Client needs category: Safe, effective care environment

Client needs subcategory: Safety and infection control

Cognitive level: Analysis

10. A client is preparing to undergo abdominal para-centesis. After explaining the procedure to the client, what should the nurse instruct the client to do to minimize the risk of accidental injury from the needle?

ANSWER: Void

Rationale: The nurse should instruct the client to void before the procedure to minimize the risk of accidental bladder injury from the needle or trocar and cannula.

Nursing process step: Implementation

Client needs category: Safe, effective care environment

Client needs subcategory: Safety and infection control

Cognitive level: Application

---

11. Locate the abdominal quadrant where the nurse would expect to palpate the liver.

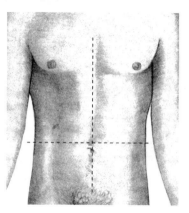

ANSWER:

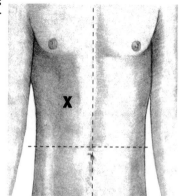

Rationale: The liver is located in the right upper abdominal quadrant.

Nursing process step: Data collection

Client needs category: Health promotion and maintenance

Client needs subcategory: Prevention and early detection of disease

Cognitive level: Knowledge

1. A client who was transferred from a long-term care facility is admitted with dehydration and pneumonia. During an assessment, the nurse observes partial-thickness skin loss involving the epidermis and dermis on the client's sacrum. As what stage pressure ulcer should the nurse document this finding?

ANSWER: 2

Rationale: The nurse should document her finding as a stage 2 pressure ulcer, which is characterized by partial-thickness skin loss involving the epidermis, dermis, or both.

Nursing process step: Data collection

Client needs category: Physiological integrity

Client needs subcategory: Basic care and comfort

Cognitive level: Knowledge

2. Which nursing interventions are effective in preventing pressure ulcers?

Select all that apply:

☑ **A.** Clean the skin with warm water and a mild cleaning agent; then apply a moisturizer.

☐ **B.** When turning the client, slide him and avoid lifting him.

☐ **C.** Avoid raising the head of the bed more than 90 degrees.

☐ **D.** Turn and reposition the client every 1 to 2 hours unless contraindicated.

☐ **E.** If the client uses a wheelchair, seat him on a rubber or plastic doughnut.

☑ **F.** Use pillows to position the client and increase his comfort.

ANSWER: A, D, F

Rationale: Nursing interventions that are effective in preventing pressure ulcers include cleaning the skin with warm water and a mild cleaning agent, and then applying a moisturizer; lifting — rather than sliding — the client when turning him to reduce friction and shear; avoiding raising the head of the bed more than 30 degrees, except for brief periods; repositioning and turning the client every 1 to 2 hours unless contraindicated; and using pillows to position the client and increase his comfort. If the client uses a wheelchair, the nurse should offer a pressure-relieving cushion as appropriate. She should not seat him on a rubber or plastic doughnut because these devices can increase localized pressure at vulnerable points.

Nursing process step: Implementation

Client needs category: Safe, effective care environment

Client needs subcategory: Safety and infection control

Cognitive level: Application

3. A 42-year-old client comes to the clinic and states that she has been experiencing fever and malaise for the past 4 days. She presents with severe, deep pain and small, red, nodular skin lesions around her thorax. The physician diagnoses her with shingles. Based on this diagnosis, the nurse should instruct the client to avoid close contact with individuals who haven't had a specific type of contagious disease until the eruption has resolved. What is this contagious disease?

_____

ANSWER: Chickenpox

Rationale: Shingles, also called herpes zoster, is an acute unilateral and segmental inflammation of the dorsal root ganglia. It's caused by infection with the herpesvirus varicella-zoster, the same virus that causes chickenpox. Therefore, to prevent the spread of infection, the nurse should warn the client to avoid close contact with individuals who haven't had chickenpox until the eruption has resolved.

Nursing process step: Planning

Client needs category: Safe, effective care environment

Client needs subcategory: Safety and infection control

Cognitive level: Application

---

4. Which instructions should be included in the teaching plan of a 19-year-old client with acne vulgaris who's prescribed tretinoin, benzoyl peroxide, and tetracycline?

Select all that apply:

☐ **A.** Expect your skin to look red and start to peel after treatment.

☐ **B.** Take tetracycline on an empty stomach.

☐ **C.** Use tretinoin and benzoyl peroxide together in the morning and at night.

☐ **D.** Maintain the prescribed treatment because it is more likely to improve acne than a strict diet and fanatic scrubbing with soap and water.

☐ **E.** Apply tretinoin at least 30 minutes after washing the face and at bedtime.

☐ **F.** Avoid exposure to sunlight and don't use a sunscreen.

ANSWER: B, D

Rationale: The nurse should instruct the client receiving tretinoin that his skin should look pink and dry after treatment. If the skin appears red or starts to peel, the preparation may have to be weakened or applied less often. The client should be instructed to take tetracycline on an empty stomach. Because the prescribed regimen includes tretinoin and benzoyl peroxide, the nurse should instruct the client to use one preparation in the morning and the other at night. Tretinoin should be applied 30 minutes after washing the face and at least 1 hour before bedtime. The nurse should also make sure that the client understands that the prescribed treatment is more likely to improve acne than are a strict diet and fanatic scrubbing with soap and water. The nurse should advise the client to avoid exposure to sunlight or to use a sunscreen.

Nursing process step: Planning

Client needs category: Physiological integrity

Client needs subcategory: Pharmacological therapies

Cognitive level: Application

5. Despite conventional treatment, a client's psoriasis has worsened. His physician prescribes methotrexate 25 mg by mouth as a single weekly dose. The pharmacy dispenses 2.5-mg scored tablets. How many tablets should the nurse instruct the client to consume to achieve the prescribed dose?

_____

Rationale: The correct formula to calculate a drug dose is:

dose on hand/quantity on hand = dose desired/X.

The physician prescribes 25 mg, which is the dose desired. The pharmacy dispenses 2.5-mg tablets, which is the dose on hand. Therefore:

2.5 mg/1 tablet = 25 mg/X tablets. X = 10 tablets.

Nursing process step: Planning

Client needs category: Physiological integrity

Client needs subcategory: Pharmacological therapies

Cognitive level: Application

---

6. A 35-year-old client is brought to the emergency department with second- and third-degree burns over 15% of his body. His admission vital signs are: blood pressure 100/50 mm Hg, heart rate 130 beats/minute, and respiratory rate 26 breaths/minute. Which nursing interventions are appropriate for this client?

Select all that apply:

☐ **A.** Clean the burns with hydrogen peroxide.

☐ **B.** Cover the burns with saline-soaked towels.

☑ **C.** Begin an I.V. infusion of lactated Ringer's solution.

☐ **D.** Place ice directly on the burn areas.

☑ **E.** Administer 6 mg of morphine I.V.

☑ **F.** Administer tetanus prophylaxis, as ordered.

Answer: C, E, F

Rationale: Immediate interventions for this client should aim to stop the burning and relieve the pain. The nurse should begin I.V. therapy with a crystalloid such as lactated Ringer's solution to prevent hypovolemic shock and to maintain cardiac output. She should administer pain medication, as ordered. Typically, 2 to 25 mg of morphine or 5 to 15 mg of meperidine are administered I.V. in small increments. Tetanus prophylaxis should be administered, as ordered. The nurse shouldn't use hydrogen peroxide or povidone-iodine solution to clean the burns because these preparations can further damage tissue. The nurse should avoid the use of saline-soaked towels because they may lead to hypothermia. Ice should not be placed directly on burn wounds because the cold may cause further thermal damage.

Nursing process step: Implementation

Client needs category: Physiological integrity

Client needs subcategory: Physiological adaptation

Cognitive level: Application

1. The nurse is assisting in planning care for a client with human immunodeficiency virus (HIV). Which statement by the nurse indicates her understanding of HIV transmission?

Select all that apply:

☐ **A.** "I will wear a gown, mask, and gloves with all client contact."

☐ **B.** "I don't need to wear any personal protective equipment due to decreased risk of occupational exposure."

☐ **C.** "I will wear a mask if the client has a cough caused by an upper respiratory infection."

☑ **D.** "I will wear a mask, gown, and gloves when splashing of bodily fluids is likely."

☑ **E.** "I will wash my hands after client care."

ANSWER: D AND E

Rationale: Standard precautions include wearing gloves for any known or anticipated contact with blood, body fluids, tissue, mucous membranes, and nonintact skin. If the task or procedure may result in splashing or splattering of blood or body fluids to the face, the nurse should wear a mask and goggles or face shield. If the task or procedure may result in splashing or splattering of blood or body fluids, the nurse should wear a fluid-resistant gown or apron. The nurse should wash her hands before and after client care and after removing gloves. A gown, mask, and gloves aren't necessary for all client care unless contact with bodily fluids, tissue, mucous membranes, and nonintact skin is expected. Nurses have an increased, not decreased, risk of occupational exposure to blood-borne pathogens. HIV is not transmitted in sputum unless blood is present.

Nursing process step: Planning

Client needs category: Safe, effective care environment

Client needs subcategory: Safety and infection control

Cognitive level: Application

2. A client has undergone total gastrectomy due to stomach cancer. Which type of anemia is the client at risk for?

ANSWER: Pernicious

Rationale: After gastrectomy, the client no longer has the intrinsic factor available to promote vitamin B12 absorption in the GI tract. As a result, deoxyribonucleic acid synthesis is inhibited, resulting in defective maturation of red blood cells.

Nursing process step: Implementation

Client needs category: Physiological integrity

Client needs subcategory: Physiological adaptation

Cognitive level: Application

3. The nurse is preparing a client with systemic lupus erythematosus (SLE) for discharge. Which instructions should the nurse include in the teaching plan?

Select all that apply:

☑ **A.** Stay out of direct sunlight.

☐ **B.** Refrain from limiting activity between flare-ups.

☑ **C.** Monitor body temperature.

☑ **D.** Taper the corticosteroid dosage as order by the physician when symptoms are under control.

☐ **E.** Apply cold packs to relieve joint pain and stiffness.

ANSWER: A, C, D

Rationale: The client with SLE should stay out of direct sunlight and avoid other sources of ultraviolet light because they may precipitate severe skin reactions and exacerbate the disease. The client should monitor his temperature, because fever can signal an exacerbation, which he should report to the physician. Corticosteroids must be tapered gradually once symptoms are relieved because they can suppress the function of the adrenal glands. Stopping corticosteroids abruptly can cause adrenal insufficiency, a potentially life-threatening condition. Fatigue can cause a flare-up of SLE; encourage clients to pace activities and plan for rest periods. The client should apply heat, not cold, to relieve joint pain. Cold packs may aggravate Raynaud's phenomenon, which commonly occurs in clients with SLE.

Nursing process step: Planning

Client needs category: Physiological integrity

Client needs subcategory: Reduction of risk potential

Cognitive level: Application

---

4. A client who is a carrier for hemophilia has just given birth to a baby boy. The father of the neonate does not have hemophilia. What percent chance does the mother have of transmitting the gene to her son?

ANSWER: 50

Rationale: Hemophilia is inherited as an X-linked recessive trait. This means that a female carrier has a 50% chance of transmitting the gene to her son.

Nursing process step: Data collection

Client needs category: Health promotion and maintenance

Client needs subcategory: Prevention and early detection of disease

Cognitive level: Analysis

5. The nurse is preparing a client for bone marrow biopsy to rule out leukemia. The nurse explains that the sample will be taken from the anterior iliac crest. Identify this area.

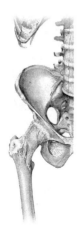

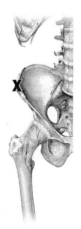

Rationale: A bone marrow biopsy may be taken from the anterior or posterior iliac crests, sternum, vertebral spinous process, rib, or tibia.

Nursing process step: Implementation

Client needs category: Physiological integrity

Client needs subcategory: Physiological adaptation

Cognitive level: Comprehension

---

6. A client with leukemia has enlarged lymph nodes, liver, and spleen. Identify the quadrant of the abdomen where the nurse would palpate the enlarged spleen.

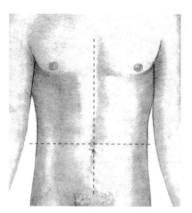

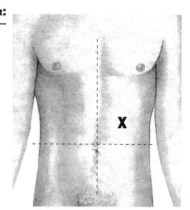

Rationale: The spleen is located in the left upper quadrant of the abdomen, posterior to the stomach.

Nursing process step: Data collection

Client needs category: Physiological integrity

Client needs subcategory: Physiological adaptation

Cognitive level: Comprehension

1. A male client is admitted to the hospital with weight loss, lethargy, and hypotension. The client's skin is bronze, despite efforts to protect his skin from the sun. After reviewing the client's past medical history, the nurse notes that the client was in a motor vehicle accident that required emergency surgery to reduce long-term kidney damage. The adrenal glands were not spared. What endocrine malfunction is this client experiencing?

_____

ANSWER: Addison's disease

Rationale: Addison's disease occurs when the adrenal glands malfunction, leading to low levels of mineralocorticoids, glucocorticoids, and androgens in the blood. A person can develop this condition after trauma to or surgical removal of the glands. Signs and symptoms of this disease include anorexia, diarrhea, nausea, bronzed skin, weakness, lethargy, and hypotension.

Nursing process step: Data collection

Client needs category: Physiological integrity

Client needs subcategory: Physiological adaptation

Cognitive level: Comprehension

2. A businesswoman comes into the clinic with a progressively enlarging neck. The client has been in a foreign country during the past 3 months and mentions that she couldn't eat that country's cuisine because of gastric intolerance. The client also states that she becomes dizzy when she lifts her arms to do normal household chores and when she's dressing. What endocrine disorder would you expect the physician to diagnose?

_____

ANSWER: Goiter

Rationale: A goiter can result from inadequate dietary intake of iodine associated with changes in diet or malnutrition. It's caused by insufficient thyroid gland production and depletion of glandular iodine. Signs and symptoms of this malfunction include enlargement of the thyroid gland, dizziness when raising the arms above the head, dysphagia, and respiratory distress.

Nursing process step: Data collection

Client needs category: Physiological integrity

Client needs subcategory: Physiological adaptation

Cognitive level: Comprehension

3. A client with type 1 diabetes mellitus has an increased heart rate and is complaining of light-headedness, sweating, and palpitations. What complication should the nurse suspect?

_____

ANSWER: Hypoglycemia

Rationale: Signs and symptoms of hypoglycemia include sweating, tremor, tachycardia, palpitations, nervousness, light-headedness, and hunger.

Nursing process step: Data collection

Client needs category: Physiological integrity

Client needs subcategory: Physiological adaptation

Cognitive level: Application

4. After falling off a ladder and suffering a brain injury, a client develops syndrome of inappropriate antidiuretic hormone (SIADH). Which of the following findings indicate the effectiveness of the treatment he is receiving?

Select all that apply:

☑ **A.** Decrease in body weight

☐ **B.** Rise in blood pressure and drop in heart rate

☐ **C.** Absence of wheezes in the lungs

☐ **D.** Increased urine output

☑ **E.** Decreased urine osmolarity

ANSWER: A, D, E

Rationale: SIADH is an abnormality in which there is an abundance of the antidiuretic hormone. The predominant feature is water retention, as well as oliguria, edema, and weight gain. Evidence of successful treatment includes a reduction in weight, an increase in urine output, and a decrease in the urine's concentration (urine osmolarity).

Nursing process step: Evaluation

Client needs category: Physiological integrity

Client needs subcategory: Physiological adaptation

Cognitive level: Analysis

5. A 48-year-old female client is seen in the clinic for newly diagnosed hypothyroidism. Which of the following topics should the nurse include in a client teaching plan?

Select all that apply:

☐ **A.** High-protein, high-calorie diet

☑ **B.** High-fiber, low-calorie diet

☐ **C.** Plan for a thyroidectomy

☑ **D.** Use of stool softeners

☑ **E.** Thyroid hormone replacements

☐ **F.** Review of the procedure for thyroid radiation therapy

ANSWER: B, D, E

Rationale: The treatment for hypothyroidism includes a high-fiber, low-calorie diet because weight gain and constipation are two symptoms of the disorder. Stool softeners are prescribed to prevent constipation, and thyroid hormone replacements are needed to supplement the underfunctioning thyroid gland. A high-protein, high-calorie diet is commonly used for clients with hyperthyroidism, along with thyroidectomy or irradiation of the thyroid gland.

Nursing process step: Planning

Client needs category: Physiological integrity

Client needs subcategory: Reduction of risk potential

Cognitive level: Application

---

6. A client who has been seen in the clinic is scheduled for an outpatient thyroid scan in 2 weeks. Which of the following instructions should the nurse include in her client teaching so that this client is prepared?

Select all that apply:

☐ **A.** Stop using iodized salt or iodized salt substitutes 1 week before the scan.

☐ **B.** Stop eating seafood 1 week before the scan.

☐ **C.** Don't consume any food or fluids after midnight on the night before the scan.

☐ **D.** Don't take prescribed thyroid medication on the day of the scan.

☐ **E.** Don't take prescribed thyroid medication until the results of the scan are known.

☐ **F.** Maintain bed rest for 24 hours after the scan.

ANSWER: A, B, D

Rationale: A thyroid scan visualizes the distribution of radioactive dye in the thyroid gland. Interventions before the scan include stopping the ingestion of iodine, which is found in iodized salt, salt substitutes, and seafood. The client should also be instructed not to take any medication that would interfere with the scan. The client doesn't have to refrain from consuming food or fluids after midnight if the scan is done on an outpatient basis. The radioactive dye is administered intravenously. Routinely prescribed medications can be taken after the scan. Bed rest is maintained with a thyroid biopsy, not a scan.

Nursing process step: Implementation

Client needs category: Physiological integrity

Client needs subcategory: Reduction of risk potential

Cognitive level: Application

7. A client is admitted to the hospital with signs and symptoms of diabetes mellitus. Which of the following findings is the nurse most likely to observe in this client?

Select all that apply:

☑ **A.** Excessive thirst

☐ **B.** Weight gain

☐ **C.** Constipation

☑ **D.** Excessive hunger

☐ **E.** Urine retention

☑ **F.** Frequent, high-volume urination

ANSWER: A, D, F

Rationale: Classic signs of diabetes mellitus include polydipsia (excessive thirst), polyphagia (excessive hunger), and polyuria (excessive urination). Because the body is starving from the lack of glucose the cells are using for energy, the client has weight loss, not weight gain. Clients with diabetes mellitus usually don't present with constipation.

Nursing process step: Data collection

Client needs category: Health promotion and maintenance

Client needs subcategory: Prevention and early detection of disease

Cognitive level: Analysis

---

8. A 56-year-old female client is being discharged after having a thyroidectomy. Which of the following discharge instructions are appropriate for this client?

Select all that apply:

☐ **A.** Report any signs and symptoms of hypoglycemia.

☑ **B.** Take thyroid replacement medication, as ordered.

☐ **C.** Watch for changes in body functioning, such as lethargy, restlessness, sensitivity to cold, and dry skin. Report them to the physician.

☐ **D.** Recognize the signs of dehydration.

☐ **E.** Avoid over-the-counter medications.

☐ **F.** Carry injectable dexamethasone at all times.

ANSWER: B, C

Rationale: After removal of the thyroid gland, the client needs to take thyroid replacement medication. The client needs to report to the physician changes in body functioning, such as lethargy, restlessness, cold sensitivity, and dry skin, because they may indicate the need to increase the medication dose. The thyroid gland doesn't regulate the serum glucose level; therefore, the client wouldn't need to recognize the signs and symptoms of hypoglycemia. Dehydration is seen in diabetes insipidus. A client with Addison's disease should avoid over-the-counter medications and carry injectable dexamethasone.

Nursing process step: Implementation

Client needs category: Physiological integrity

Client needs subcategory: Physiological adaptation

Cognitive level: Application

9. A client is seen in the clinic with suspected parathormone (PTH) deficiency. Part of the diagnosis of this condition includes the analysis of serum electrolyte levels. The levels of which of the following electrolytes would the nurse expect to be abnormal in a client with PTH deficiency?

Select all that apply:

☐ **A.** Sodium

☐ **B.** Potassium

☑ **C.** Calcium

☐ **D.** Chloride

☐ **E.** Glucose

☑ **F.** Phosphorus

ANSWER: C, F

Rationale: A client with PTH deficiency has abnormal serum calcium and phosphorus levels because PTH regulates these two electrolytes. PTH deficiency doesn't affect sodium, potassium, chloride, or glucose.

Nursing process step: Evaluation

Client needs category: Health promotion and maintenance

Client needs subcategory: Prevention and early detection of disease

Cognitive level: Analysis

---

10. A client is placed on hypocalcemia precautions after removal of the parathyroid gland for cancer. The nurse should observe the client for which of the following symptoms?

Select all that apply:

☐ **A.** Numbness

☐ **B.** Aphasia

☐ **C.** Tingling

☐ **D.** Muscle twitching and spasms

☐ **E.** Polyuria

☐ **F.** Polydipsia

ANSWER: A, C, D

Rationale: When the parathyroid gland is removed, the body may not produce enough parathyroid hormone to regulate calcium and phosphorus levels. The symptoms of hypocalcemia include peripheral numbness, tingling, and muscle spasms. Aphasia isn't a symptom of calcium depletion. Polyuria and polydipsia are symptoms of diabetes mellitus.

Nursing process step: Data collection

Client needs category: Physiological integrity

Client needs subcategory: Reduction of risk potential

Cognitive level: Analysis

11. A 45-year-old female client is admitted to the hospital with Cushing's syndrome. Which of the following nursing interventions are appropriate for this client?

Select all that apply:

☑ **A.** Assess for peripheral edema.

☐ **B.** Stress the need for a high-calorie, high-carbohydrate diet.

☐ **C.** Measure intake and output.

☑ **D.** Encourage oral fluid intake.

☑ **E.** Weigh the client daily.

☐ **F.** Instruct the client to avoid foods high in potassium.

ANSWER: A, C, E

Rationale: Because weight gain and edema are common symptoms of Cushing's syndrome, appropriate interventions include assessing for peripheral edema, measuring intake and output, and weighing the client daily. A low-calorie, low-carbohydrate, high-protein diet is ordered for a client with this disorder. Fluid restriction is often prescribed as well. Treatment of Cushing's syndrome includes the administration of potassium replacements; therefore, restricting foods high in potassium wouldn't be appropriate.

Nursing process step: Implementation

Client needs category: Physiological integrity

Client needs subcategory: Physiological adaptation

Cognitive level: Application

---

12. A client with type 2 diabetes mellitus needs instruction on proper foot care. Which of the following instructions should the nurse include in client teaching?

Select all that apply:

☐ **A.** Be sure to use scissors to trim toenails.

☑ **B.** Wear cotton socks.

☐ **C.** Apply foot powder after bathing.

☐ **D.** Go barefoot only when you know your home environment.

☐ **E.** See a podiatrist regularly to have your feet checked.

☑ **F.** Wear loose-fitting shoes.

ANSWER: B, C, E

Rationale: Foot care for a client with diabetes mellitus includes keeping the feet dry with the application of foot powder and wearing cotton socks to absorb moisture. The client should have a podiatrist check his feet regularly to detect problems early. To prevent injury to the feet, the client should be instructed not to cut his toenails with scissors, walk barefoot, or wear loose-fitting shoes.

Nursing process step: Implementation

Client needs category: Physiological integrity

Client needs subcategory: Reduction of risk potential

Cognitive level: Application

1. A 72-year-old female client reports that she has lost an inch in height over the past 15 years. The nurse recognizes this as a sign of which musculoskeletal disorder?

_____

Answer: Osteoporosis

Rationale: The client with osteoporosis is typically a postmenopausal woman who may report that she has had a gradual loss of height since menopause.

Nursing process step: Implementation

Client needs category: Health promotion and maintenance

Client needs subcategory: Prevention and early detection of disease

Cognitive level: Comprehension

2. A client is preparing for discharge from the hospital after undergoing an above-the-knee amputation. Which of the following instructions should the nurse include in the teaching plan for this client?

Select all that apply:

☐ **A.** Massage the stump away from the suture line.

☐ **B.** Avoid using heat application to ease pain.

☐ **C.** Report twitching, spasms, or phantom limb pain immediately.

☐ **D.** Avoid exposing the skin around the stump to excessive perspiration.

☐ **E.** Be sure to perform the prescribed exercises.

☐ **F.** Rub the stump with a dry washcloth for 4 minutes three times per day if the stump is sensitive to touch.

Answer: D, E, F

Rationale: The nurse should advise the client to avoid exposing the skin around the stump to excessive perspiration, which can be irritating. She should tell him to perform prescribed exercises to help minimize complications. In addition, the nurse should tell the client that if the stump is sensitive to touch, he should rub the stump with a dry washcloth for 4 minutes three times per day. The nurse should tell the client to massage the stump toward — not away from — the suture line to mobilize the scar and to prevent its adherence to bone. The client may experience twitching, spasms, or phantom limb pain while his muscles adjust to the amputation. This is a normal reaction and doesn't need to be reported. The nurse should advise the client that he can ease these symptoms with heat, massage, or gentle pressure.

Nursing process step: Planning

Client needs category: Physiological integrity

Client needs subcategory: Reduction of risk potential

Cognitive level: Application

3. A client is scheduled for a laminectomy of L1-L2. The nurse is teaching the client about the procedure. Identify the area that the nurse explains will be involved in this client's surgery.

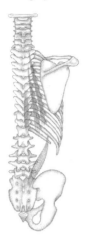

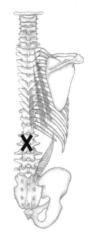

Rationale: In laminectomy, one or more of the bony laminae that cover the vertebrae are removed. There are five lumbar vertebrae, so the nurse can count up from the sacrum to locate L1-L2. Vertebrae are numbered from top to bottom, with L5 being closest to the sacrum.

Nursing process step: Implementation

Client needs category: Physiological integrity

Client needs subcategory: Physiologic adaptation

Cognitive level: Comprehension

---

4. A client is diagnosed with gout. Which of the following foods should the nurse instruct the client to avoid?

Select all that apply:

☐ **A.** Green leafy vegetables

☐ **B.** Liver

☐ **C.** Cod

☐ **D.** Chocolate

☑ **E.** Sardines

☐ **F.** Eggs

☐ **G.** Whole milk

ANSWER: B, C, E

Rationale: The client with gout should avoid foods that are high in purines, such as liver, cod, and sardines. Other foods that should be avoided include anchovies, kidneys, sweetbreads, lentils, and alcoholic beverages, especially beer and wine. Green leafy vegetables, chocolate, eggs, and whole milk are not high in purines and, therefore, are not restricted in the diet of a client with gout.

Nursing process step: Implementation

Client needs category: Physiological integrity

Client needs subcategory: Basic care and comfort

Cognitive level: Application

5. A client is about to undergo total hip replacement surgery. Before the surgery, the nurse conducts a pre-operative teaching session with him. The nurse can tell that her teaching her been effective when the client verbalizes the importance of avoiding which of the following actions?

Select all that apply:

☐ **A.** Keeping the legs apart while lying in bed

☐ **B.** Periodically tightening the leg muscles

☐ **C.** Internally rotating the feet

☐ **D.** Bending to pick items up from the floor

☐ **E.** Sleeping in a side-lying position

ANSWER: C, D

Rationale: After hip replacement surgery, the client should avoid internally rotating his feet and bending more than 90 degrees. These activities can compromise the hip joint. The client should lie with his legs abducted. Leg-strengthening exercises, such as periodically tightening the leg muscles, are recommended to maintain muscle strength and reduce the risk of thrombus formation. A side-lying position is acceptable; however, some physicians restrict lying on the operative side.

Nursing process step: Evaluation

Client needs category: Physiological integrity

Client needs subcategory: Reduction of risk potential

Cognitive level: Analysis

---

6. A client who was involved in a motor vehicle accident has a fractured femur. The nurse caring for the client identifies *Acute pain* as one of the nursing diagnoses in his care plan. Which of the following nursing interventions are appropriate?

Select all that apply:

☐ **A.** Tell the client which pain management option to use.

☐ **B.** Encourage the client to use as little pain medication as possible to avoid addiction.

☐ **C.** Explain that pain management should leave the client pain-free.

☐ **D.** Avoid alternative and supplementary pain control techniques.

☑ **E.** Assess the client's perception of pain.

☑ **F.** Ask the client about methods he previously used to alleviate pain.

ANSWER: E, F

Rationale: The nurse should begin by assessing the client's perception of pain, including characteristics, and methods he previously found effective in managing pain. These interventions provide a baseline from which the nurse can plan interventions and evaluate their success. The nurse should allow the client to decide which pain control management techniques to use to help increase his self-esteem. Analgesics should be administered as needed to relieve pain. Addiction shouldn't be a concern at this time. After receiving analgesics, the client should indicate that he feels more comfortable, by reporting pain as a score of 3 or less on a scale of 0 to 10 (0 being without pain). Being completely pain-free isn't a realistic expectation. The nurse should teach the client alternative and supplementary pain control techniques, such as imagery, distraction, and heat and cold application. These techniques provide the client with options for dealing with pain.

Nursing process step: Implementation

Client needs category: Physiological integrity

Client needs subcategory: Basic care and comfort

Cognitive level: Application

7. An elderly client fractured the neck of his femur in a fall. The nurse is using an illustration to explain to the family where the fracture occurred. Identify the area that the nurse would point out to the family as the site of the fracture.

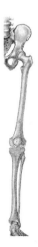

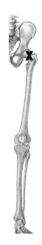

Rationale: The neck of the femur connects the round ball head of the femur to the shaft.

Nursing process step: Implementation

Client needs category: Physiological integrity

Client needs subcategory: Physiologic adaptation

Cognitive level: Comprehension

---

8. The nurse is assisting a client with range-of-motion exercises. The nurse moves the client's leg out and away from the midline of the body. What term does the nurse use to document this movement?

_____

ANSWER: Abduction

Rationale: Movement away from the body or midline is called abduction. Movement toward the midline is called adduction.

Nursing process step: Implementation

Client needs category: Physiological integrity

Client needs subcategory: Basic care and comfort

Cognitive level: Comprehension

1. A client with active pulmonary tuberculosis is treated with streptomycin. Which of the five senses should the nurse monitor for evidence of damage caused by the streptomycin?

ANSWER: Hearing

Rationale: Streptomycin, an aminoglycoside, can damage the eighth cranial nerve (acoustic nerve), resulting in hearing loss, roaring noises, and fullness in the ears.

Nursing process step: Data collection

Client needs category: Physiological integrity

Client needs subcategory: Reduction of risk potential

Cognitive level: Comprehension

---

2. The nurse is caring for a client who is being evaluated for a head injury. The physician decides to perform an ice water caloric test to determine if the brain stem is intact. Into which structure should the nurse expect the physician to inject the ice water?

ANSWER: Ear

Rationale: In the ice water caloric test, a syringe of ice water is injected into the client's ear to evaluate eye response. A client with a brain injury that involves the vestibular branch of the eighth cranial nerve (acoustic nerve) won't exhibit the normal eye movements associated with caloric testing.

Nursing process step: Data collection

Client needs category: Physiological integrity

Client needs subcategory: Reduction of risk potential

Cognitive level: Knowledge

3. The nurse is observing a client with cerebral edema for evidence of increasing intracranial pressure. She monitors his blood pressure for signs of widening pulse pressure. His current blood pressure is 170/80 mm Hg. What is the client's pulse pressure?

_____

ANSWER: 90

Rationale: Pulse pressure is the difference between the systolic blood pressure and the diastolic blood pressure. For this client, pulse pressure = 170 − 80 = 90.

Nursing process step: Data collection

Client needs category: Physiological integrity

Client needs subcategory: Reduction of risk potential

Cognitive level: Application

---

4. A client is quadriplegic secondary to a spinal cord injury from a motor vehicle accident. At which segment of the spinal cord did the injury most likely occur?

_____

ANSWER: Cervical

Rationale: Quadriplegia occurs as a result of injury to the cervical segment of the spinal cord.

Nursing process step: Data collection

Client needs category: Physiological integrity

Client needs subcategory: Physiological adaptation

Cognitive level: Comprehension

5. A nurse examines a client's level of responsiveness. She finds that the client opens his eyes spontaneously, obeys verbal commands, and is oriented to time, place, and person. What is the client's Glasgow Coma Scale score?

Glasgow Coma Scale

Eye opening response

Opens spontaneously = 4
Opens to verbal command = 3
Opens to pain = 2
No response = 1

4 + 6 + 5

Best motor response

Obeys verbal commands = 6
Localizes painful stimuli = 5
Flexion-withdrawal = 4
Flexion-abnormal (decorticate rigidity) = 3
Extension (decerebrate rigidity) = 1

Best verbal response

Oriented and converses = 5
Disoriented and converses = 4
Inappropriate words = 3
Incomprehensible sounds = 2
No response = 1

ANSWER: 15

Rationale: The score for spontaneous eye opening is 4; obeying verbal commands, 6; and orientation to time, place and person, 5. The total Glasgow Coma Scale score for this client is 15.

Nursing process step: Data collection

Client needs category: Physiological integrity

Client needs subcategory: Physiological adaptation

Cognitive level: Comprehension

---

6. A client who had a massive stroke exhibits the posture illustrated. The nurse documents what type of posture?

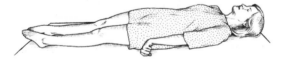

ANSWER: Decerebrate

Rationale: Decerebrate posture, which results from damage to the upper brain stem, is characterized by adduction and extension of the arms. These findings are accompanied by wrist pronation, finger flexion, and stiff extension of the legs with plantar flexion of the feet.

Nursing process step: Data collection

Client needs category: Physiological integrity

Client needs subcategory: Physiological adaptation

Cognitive level: Knowledge

7. A client with a history of epilepsy is admitted to the medical-surgical unit. While assisting the client from the bathroom, the nurse observes the start of a tonic-clonic seizure. Which nursing interventions are appropriate for this client?

Select all that apply:

☑ **A.** Assist the client to the floor.

☑ **B.** Turn the client to his side.

☑ **C.** Place a pillow under the client's head.

☐ **D.** Give the prescribed dose of oral phenytoin (Dilantin).

☐ **E.** Insert an oral suction device to remove secretions in the mouth.

ANSWER: A, B, C

Rationale: During a seizure, the nurse should assist the client to the floor to reduce the risk of falling and turn the client on his side to help clear the mouth of oral secretions. If available, it's appropriate to place a pillow under the client's head to protect him from injury. It's inappropriate to introduce anything into the mouth during a seizure because of the risk of choking or compromising the airway; therefore, oral medications and suction devices shouldn't be used.

Nursing process step: Implementation

Client needs category: Physiological integrity

Client needs subcategory: Reduction of risk potential

Cognitive level: Application

---

8. The nurse is assigned to care for a client with early stage Alzheimer's disease. Which nursing interventions should be included in the client's care plan?

Select all that apply:

☐ **A.** Make frequent changes in the client's routine.

☐ **B.** Engage the client in complex discussions to improve memory.

☑ **C.** Furnish the client's environment with familiar possessions.

☑ **D.** Assist the client with activities of daily living (ADLs) as necessary.

☑ **E.** Assign tasks in simple steps.

ANSWER: C, D, E

Rationale: A client with Alzheimer's disease experiences progressive deterioration in cognitive functioning. Familiar possessions may help to orient the client. The client should be encouraged to perform ADLs as much as possible but may need assistance with certain activities. Using a step-by-step approach helps the client complete tasks independently. A client with Alzheimer's disease functions best with consistent routines. Complex discussions don't improve the memory of a client with Alzheimer's disease.

Nursing process step: Planning

Client needs category: Psychosocial integrity

Client needs subcategory: Psychosocial adaptation

Cognitive level: Application

9. A client is admitted to the medical-surgical unit after undergoing intracranial surgery to remove a tumor from the left cerebral hemisphere. Which nursing interventions are appropriate for the client's postoperative care?

Select all that apply:

☐ **A.** Place a pillow under the client's head so that his neck is flexed.

☐ **B.** Turn the client on his right side.

☐ **C.** Place pillows under the client's legs to promote hip flexion and venous return.

☐ **D.** Maintain the client in the supine position.

☐ **E.** Apply a soft collar to keep the client's neck in a neutral position.

Rationale: The client should be turned on his right side because lying on the left side would cause the brain to shift into the space previously occupied by the tumor. A soft collar keeps the neck in a neutral position, allowing for adequate perfusion and venous drainage of the brain. Placing a pillow under the head flexes the neck and impairs circulation to the brain. Flexion of the hip increases intracranial pressure and, therefore, is contraindicated. Exclusive use of the supine position isn't indicated.

Nursing process step: Implementation

Client needs category: Physiological integrity

Client needs subcategory: Reduction of risk potential

Cognitive level: Application

---

10. The nurse is planning care for a client with multiple sclerosis. Which problems should the nurse expect the client to experience?

Select all that apply:

☑ **A.** Visual disturbances

☐ **B.** Coagulation abnormalities

☑ **C.** Balance problems

☐ **D.** Immunity compromise

☑ **E.** Mood disorders

ANSWER: A, C, E

Rationale: Multiple sclerosis, a neuromuscular disorder, may cause visual disturbances, balance problems, and mood disorders. Multiple sclerosis doesn't cause coagulation abnormalities or immunity problems.

Nursing process step: Planning

Client needs category: Physiological integrity

Client needs subcategory: Reduction of risk potential

Cognitive level: Application

11. The nurse is teaching a client with trigeminal neuralgia how to minimize pain episodes. Which comments by the client indicate that he understands the instructions?

Select all that apply:

- ☐ **A.** "I'll eat food that is very hot."
- ☑ **B.** "I'll try to chew my food on the unaffected side."
- ☐ **C.** "I can wash my face with cold water."
- ☑ **D.** "Drinking fluids at room temperature should reduce pain."
- ☑ **E.** "If tooth brushing is too painful, I'll try to rinse my mouth instead."

ANSWER: B, D, E

Rationale: The facial pain of trigeminal neuralgia is triggered by mechanical or thermal stimuli. Chewing food on the unaffected side and rinsing the mouth rather than brushing teeth reduce mechanical stimulation. Drinking fluids at room temperature reduces thermal stimulation. Eating hot food and washing the face with cold water are likely to trigger pain.

Nursing process step: Evaluation

Client needs category: Health promotion and maintenance

Client needs subcategory: Prevention and early detection of disease

Cognitive level: Comprehension

---

12. A client is experiencing problems with balance and fine and gross motor function. Identify that area of the client's brain that's malfunctioning.

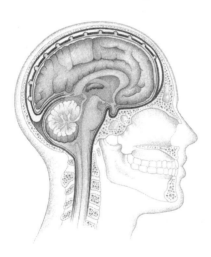

ANSWER:

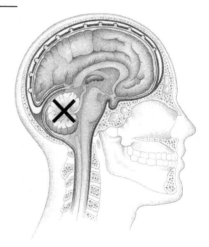

Rationale: The cerebellum is the portion of the brain that controls balance and fine and gross motor function.

Nursing process step: Data collection

Client needs category: Physiological integrity

Client needs subcategory: Reduction of risk potential

Cognitive level: Comprehension

Respiratory disorders

1. The nurse is caring for a client with pneumonia. The physician orders 600 mg of ceftriaxone (Rocephin) oral suspension to be given once per day. The medication label indicates that the strength is 125 mg/5 ml. How many milliliters of medication should the nurse pour to administer the correct dose?

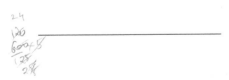

ANSWER: 24

Rationale: To calculate drug dosages, use the formula:

Dose on hand/Quantity on hand = Dose desired/X.

In this case, 125 mg/5 ml = 600 mg/X. Therefore, X = 24 ml.

Nursing process step: Implementation

Client needs category: Physiological integrity

Client needs subcategory: Pharmacological therapies

Cognitive level: Application

---

2. The nurse is caring for a client who has a chest tube connected to a three-chamber drainage system without suction. Identify the chamber that collects drainage from the client.

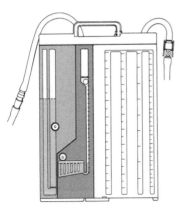

ANSWER:

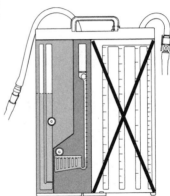

Rationale: The drainage chamber is on the right. It has three calibrated columns that show the amount of drainage collected. When the first column fills, drainage empties into the second; when the second column fills, drainage flows into the third. The water-seal chamber is located in the center. The suction-control chamber is on the left.

Nursing process step: Implementation

Client needs category: Physiological integrity

Client needs subcategory: Physiological adaptation

Cognitive level: Comprehension

3. The nurse is caring for a client with chronic obstructive pulmonary disease (COPD). When performing a physical assessment, the nurse should expect the client's chest to be what shape?

_____

Rationale: Because of chronically distended alveoli and the use of accessory muscles to assist respirations, the chest of a client with COPD develops an increased anterior-posterior diameter, making it appear barrel-shaped.

Nursing process step: Data collection

Client needs category: Physiological integrity

Client needs subcategory: Physiological adaptation

Cognitive level: Comprehension

4. A client is scheduled for a test that involves inserting a fiberoptic endoscope into the bronchi to determine a diagnosis, examine certain structures, and obtain a biopsy specimen. By what name should the nurse call this procedure when she explains it to the client?

_____

Answer: Bronchoscopy

Rationale: A bronchoscopy involves inserting a bronchoscope into the bronchi to determine a diagnosis, collect a biopsy specimen, examine structures, or remove foreign objects.

Nursing process step: Implementation

Client needs category: Physiological integrity

Client needs subcategory: Physiological adaptation

Cognitive level: Comprehension

5. The nurse administers a Mantoux test to a client to detect tuberculosis infection. What is the minimum number of hours the nurse must instruct the client to wait until he can return to have the test read?

_____

ANSWER: 48

Rationale: The Mantoux test is read no earlier than 48 hours and no later than 72 hours after administration.

Nursing process step: Implementation

Client needs category: Health promotion and maintenance

Client needs subcategory: Prevention and early detection of disease

Cognitive level: Application

---

6. The nurse is caring for a client who is scheduled for a bronchoscopy. Which interventions should the nurse perform to prepare the client for this procedure?

Select all that apply:

☑ **A.** Explain the procedure.

☐ **B.** Withhold food and fluids for 2 hours before the test.

☐ **C.** Provide a clear liquid diet for 6 to 12 hours before the test.

☑ **D.** Confirm that a signed informed consent form has been obtained.

☑ **E.** Ask the client to remove his dentures.

☑ **F.** Administer atropine and a sedative.

ANSWER: A, D, E, F

Rationale: All procedures must be explained to the client in order to obtain informed consent and to reduce anxiety. A signed informed consent form is required for all invasive procedures. Dentures need to be removed for bronchoscopy because they may become dislodged during the procedure. Atropine is administered before bronchoscopy to decrease secretions. A sedative may be given to relax the client. Food and fluids are restricted for 6 to 12 hours before the test to avoid the risk of aspiration during the procedure.

Nursing process step: Implementation

Client needs category: Physiological integrity

Client needs subcategory: Reduction of risk potential

Cognitive level: Application

7. A client has just undergone a bronchoscopy. Which nursing interventions are appropriate after this procedure?

Select all that apply:

☐ **A.** Keep the client flat for at least 2 hours.

☐ **B.** Provide sips of water to moisten the mouth.

☑ **C.** Withhold food and fluids until the gag reflex returns.

☑ **D.** Assess for hemoptysis and frank bleeding.

☐ **E.** Resume food and fluids when the client's voice returns.

☑ **F.** Monitor the client's vital signs.

ANSWER: C, D, F

Rationale: To prevent aspiration, the client shouldn't receive food or fluids until his gag reflex returns. Although a small amount of blood in the sputum is expected if a biopsy was performed, frank bleeding indicates hemorrhage and should be reported to the physician immediately. Vital signs should be monitored after the procedure because a vasovagal response may cause bradycardia, laryngospasm can affect respirations, and fever may develop within 24 hours of the procedure. To reduce the risk of aspiration, the client should be placed in a semi-Fowler's or side-lying position after the procedure until the gag reflex returns. The client doesn't lose his voice after a bronchoscopy, so voice shouldn't be used as a gauge for resuming food and fluid intake.

Nursing process step: Implementation

Client needs category: Physiological integrity

Client needs subcategory: Reduction of risk potential

Cognitive level: Application

---

8. The nurse is caring for a client with pneumonia. The nurse should expect to observe which signs and symptoms when assessing the client?

Select all that apply:

☐ **A.** Dry cough

☐ **B.** Fever

☐ **C.** Bradycardia

☐ **D.** Pericardial friction rub

☐ **E.** Use of accessory muscles during respiration

☐ **F.** Crackles or rhonchi

ANSWER: B, E, F

Rationale: The client with pneumonia may have a fever, use accessory muscles for breathing, and exhibit crackles or rhonchi on auscultation. Other signs and symptoms of pneumonia include fever, malaise, pleuritic pain, pleural friction rub, dyspnea, tachypnea, tachycardia, and a cough that produces rusty green or bloody sputum (in pneumococcal pneumonia) or yellow-green sputum (in bronchopneumonia). A dry cough, bradycardia, and a pericardial friction rub aren't manifestations of pneumonia.

Nursing process step: Data collection

Client needs category: Physiological integrity

Client needs subcategory: Physiological adaptation

Cognitive level: Application

9. The nurse is caring for a client with tuberculosis. Which precautions should the nurse take when providing care for this client?

Select all that apply:

☐ **A.** Wear gloves when handling tissues containing sputum.

☐ **B.** Wear a face mask at all times.

☐ **C.** Keep the client in strict isolation.

☐ **D.** When the client leaves the room for tests, have all people in contact with him wear a mask.

☐ **E.** Keep the client's door open to allow fresh air into the room and prevent social isolation.

☐ **F.** Wash hands after direct contact with the client or contaminated articles.

ANSWER: A, B, F

Rationale: The nurse should always wear gloves when handling items contaminated with sputum or body secretions. All staff and visitors must wear face masks when coming in contact with the client in his room; masks must be discarded before leaving the client's room. Hand washing is required after direct contact with the client or contaminated articles. Strict isolation isn't required if the client adheres to special respiratory precautions. The client, not the people in contact with him, must wear a mask when leaving the room for tests. The client should be in a negative-pressure, private room, and the door should remain closed at all times to prevent the spread of infection.

Nursing process step: Implementation

Client needs category: Safe, effective care environment

Client needs subcategory: Safety and infection control

Cognitive level: Application

---

10. A client is admitted to the progressive care unit with an arterial line for continuous measurement of systolic, diastolic, and mean blood pressures. The nurse is evaluating the waveform. Identify the area that indicates that the aortic valve has closed.

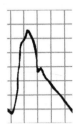

ANSWER:

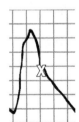

Rationale: When the pressure in the ventricle is less than the pressure in the aortic root, the aortic valve closes. This event appears as a small notch on the waveform's downside.

Nursing process step: Data collection

Client needs category: Physiological integrity

Client needs subcategory: Reduction of risk potential

Cognitive level: Comprehension

11. The nurse is about to perform nasopharyngeal suctioning on a client who recently had a cerebrovascular accident. Identify the area where the tip of the suction catheter should be placed.

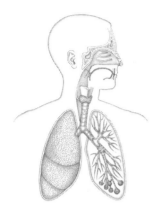

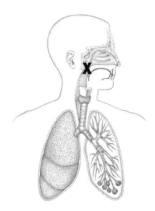

Rationale: When performing nasopharyngeal suctioning, the tip of the catheter is introduced into the naris and advanced to the pharynx. The tip remains above the posterior wall of the mouth.

Nursing process step: Implementation

Client needs category: Physiological integrity

Client needs subcategory: Physiological adaptation

Cognitive level: Application

---

12. A client is admitted with chronic obstructive pulmonary disease (COPD). Which of the following signs and symptoms are characteristic of COPD?

Select all that apply:

☐ **A.** Decreased respiratory rate

☐ **B.** Dyspnea on exertion

☐ **C.** Barrel chest

☐ **D.** Shortened expiratory phase

☐ **E.** Clubbed fingers and toes

☐ **F.** Fever

ANSWER: B, C, E

Rationale: Typical findings for clients with COPD include dyspnea on exertion, a barrel chest, and clubbed fingers and toes. Clients with COPD are usually tachypneic with a prolonged expiratory phase. Fever is not associated with COPD, unless an infection is also present.

Nursing process step: Data collection

Client needs category: Physiological integrity

Client needs subcategory: Physiological adaptation

Cognitive level: Comprehension

1. The nurse is assessing a client who has a urinary tract infection (UTI). Which of the following statements should the nurse expect the client to make?

Select all that apply:

☐ **A**. "I urinate large amounts."

☐ **B.** "I need to urinate frequently."

☐ **C.** "It burns when I urinate."

☐ **D.** "My urine smells sweet."

☐ **E.** "I need to urinate urgently."

Answer: B, C, E

Rationale: Typical assessment findings for a client with a UTI include urinary frequency, burning on urination, and urinary urgency. The client with a UTI typically reports that he voids frequently in small amounts, not large amounts. The client with a UTI complains of foul-smelling, not sweet-smelling, urine.

Nursing process step: Data collection

Client needs category: Physiological integrity

Client needs subcategory: Physiological adaptation

Cognitive level: Application

---

2. The nurse is teaching a client how to collect a 24-hour urine specimen for creatinine clearance. Which of the following directions should the nurse give the client?

Select all that apply:

☐ **A.** "Save the first voiding and record the time."

☐ **B.** "Discard the first voiding and record the time."

☐ **C.** "Clean the perineal area before each voiding."

☐ **D.** "Refrigerate the urine sample or keep it on ice."

☐ **E.** "At the end of 24 hours, void and save the urine."

☐ **F.** "At the end of 24 hours, void and discard the urine."

Answer: B, D, E

Rationale: When collecting a 24-hour urine sample, the client should void, discard the urine, and record the time. This assures that the client starts the collection period with an empty bladder. At the end of the 24-hour collection period, the client should void and save the urine. The first voiding is not used because it isn't known how long the urine has been in the bladder. The urine sample should be refrigerated or kept on ice to keep it fresh. The perineum should be cleaned before obtaining a clean-catch urine specimen for culture and sensitivity. It is not necessary to clean the perineum for a 24-hour urine sample.

Nursing process step: Implementation

Client needs category: Physiological integrity

Client needs subcategory: Reduction of risk potential

Cognitive level: Application

3. The nurse is collecting a sterile urine sample for culture and sensitivity from an indwelling urinary catheter. Identify the area on the indwelling urinary catheter where the nurse should insert the sterile syringe to obtain the urine sample.

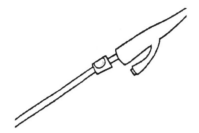

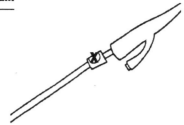

Rationale: A sterile urine specimen is obtained from an indwelling urinary catheter by clamping the catheter briefly, cleaning the rubber port with an alcohol wipe, and using a sterile syringe and needle to withdraw the urine.

Nursing process step: Implementation

Client needs category: Physiological integrity

Client needs subcategory: Reduction of risk potential

Cognitive level: Application

---

4. The nurse is completing an intake and output record for a client who is receiving continuous bladder irrigation after transurethral resection of the prostate. How many milliliters of urine should the nurse record as output for her shift if the client received 1,800 ml of normal saline irrigating solution and the output in the urine drainage bag is 2,400 ml?

ANSWER: 600

Rationale: To calculate urine output, subtract the amount of irrigation solution infused into the bladder from the total amount of fluid in the drainage bag (2,400 ml − 1,800 ml = 600 ml).

Nursing process step: Data collection

Client needs category: Physiological integrity

Client needs subcategory: Reduction of risk potential

Cognitive level: Application

5. The nurse is caring for a client with a cystostomy for urine drainage. Identify the area where the nurse should check for cystostomy placement.

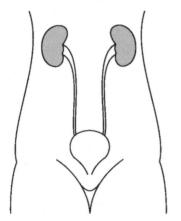

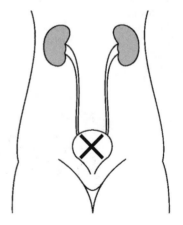

Rationale: In a cystostomy, a catheter is inserted percutaneously through the suprapubic area into the bladder.

Nursing process step: Data collection

Client needs category: Physiological integrity

Client needs subcategory: Basic care and comfort

Cognitive level: Comprehension

---

6. The nurse observes blood in the urine of a client with a urinary tract infection. What medical term should the nurse use to document this finding?

Answer: Hematuria

Rationale: Hematuria is the term used to describe blood in the urine.

Nursing process step: Data collection

Client needs category: Physiological integrity

Client needs subcategory: Reduction of risk potential

Cognitive level: Knowledge

Part 3
Maternal-infant nursing

1. A client comes to the office for her first prenatal visit. She reports that October 5 was the first day of her last menstrual period. According to Nägele's rule, what date should the nurse record as the estimated date of delivery (EDD)?

ANSWER: JULY 12

Rationale: The nurse can calculate EDD using Nägele's rule (subtract 3 months from the first day of the last menstrual period and then add 7 days). In this example, October 5 minus 3 months is July 5. Adding 7 days to July 5 makes the EDD July 12.

Nursing process step: Data collection

Client needs category: Health promotion and maintenance

Client needs subcategory: Growth and development through the life span

Cognitive level: Comprehension

2. The nurse is assisting with a prenatal assessment on a client who is 32 weeks pregnant. She performs Leopold's maneuvers and determines that the fetus is in the cephalic position. Identify where the nurse should place the Doppler to auscultate fetal heart tones.

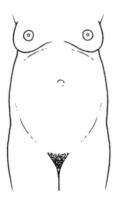

ANSWER:

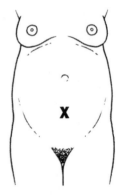

Rationale: When the fetus is in the cephalic position (head down), fetal heart tones are best auscultated midway between the symphysis pubis and the umbilicus. When the fetus is in the breech position, fetal heart tones are best heard at or above the level of the umbilicus.

Nursing process step: Data collection

Client needs category: Health promotion and maintenance

Client needs subcategory: Growth and development through the life span

Cognitive level: Analysis

3. The nurse is providing instruction to a woman who is 18 weeks pregnant. The client tells the nurse that she has felt light fluttering in her abdomen. The nurse explains that this is normal. What is the clinical term for this sensation?

_____

ANSWER: Quickening

Rationale: Quickening, which is typically described as light fluttering and is usually felt between 16 and 22 weeks' gestation, is caused by fetal movement. It is a presumptive sign of pregnancy.

Nursing process step: Implementation

Client needs category: Health promotion and maintenance

Client needs subcategory: Growth and development through the life span

Cognitive level: Comprehension

4. Which of the following nutritional instructions should the nurse provide to a 32-year-old primigravida?

Select all that apply:

- ☐ **A.** Caloric intake should be increased 300 cal/day.
- ☐ **B.** Protein intake should be increased to more than 30 g/day.
- ☐ **C.** Vitamin intake should not increase from prepregnancy requirements.
- ☐ **D.** Folic acid intake should be increased to 400 mg/day.
- ☐ **E.** Intake of all minerals, especially iron, should be increased.

ANSWER: A, B, E

Rationale: A pregnant woman should increase her caloric intake by 300 cal/day. The protein requirements (76 g/day) of a pregnant woman exceed those of a nonpregnant woman by 30 g/day. All mineral requirements, especially iron, are increased in a pregnant woman. The woman should increase her intake of all vitamins and a prenatal vitamin is usually recommended. Folic acid intake is particularly important to help prevent fetal anomalies such as neural tube defect. Intake should be increased from 400 to 800 mg/day.

Nursing process step: Planning

Client needs category: Physiological integrity

Client needs subcategory: Basic care and comfort

Cognitive level: Comprehension

5. During a prenatal screening of a client with diabetes, the nurse should keep in mind that the client is at increased risk for which of the following complications?

Select all that apply:

☐ **A.** Still birth

☐ **B.** Rh incompatibility

☐ **C.** Pregnancy-induced hypertension

☐ **D.** Placenta previa

☐ **E.** Spontaneous abortion

ANSWER: A, C, E

Rationale: Diabetic clients are at increased risk for intrauterine fetal death after 36 weeks' gestation. Gestational diabetes is also associated with an increased risk of pregnancy-induced hypertension and spontaneous abortion. The risk of Rh incompatibility and placenta previa isn't increased in the client with diabetes.

Nursing process step: Data collection

Client needs category: Health promotion and maintenance

Client needs subcategory: Prevention and early detection of disease

Cognitive level: Comprehension

---

6. A client is scheduled for amniocentesis. What should the nurse do to prepare the client for the procedure?

Select all that apply:

☐ **A.** Ask the client to void.

☐ **B.** Instruct the client to drink 1 L of fluid.

☐ **C.** Ask the client to lie on her left side.

☑ **D.** Assess fetal heart rate.

☐ **E.** Insert an I.V. catheter.

☐ **F.** Monitor maternal vital signs.

ANSWER: A, D, F

Rationale: To prepare a client for amniocentesis, the nurse should ask the client to empty her bladder to reduce the risk of bladder perforation. Prior to the procedure, the nurse should also assess fetal heart rate and maternal vital signs to establish baselines. The client should be asked to drink 1 L of fluid before transabdominal ultrasound, not amniocentesis. The client should be supine during the procedure; afterward, she should be placed on her left side to avoid supine hypotension, to promote venous return, and to ensure adequate cardiac output. I.V. access isn't necessary for this procedure.

Nursing process step: Implementation

Client needs category: Physiological integrity

Client needs subcategory: Reduction of risk potential

Cognitive level: Application

7. A client with hyperemesis gravidarum is on a clear liquid diet. Which of the following foods would be appropriate for the nurse to serve?

Select all that apply:

☐ **A.** Milk and ice chips

☐ **B.** Decaffeinated coffee and scrambled eggs

☑ **C.** Tea and gelatin

☑ **D.** Ginger ale and apple juice

☑ **E.** Cranberry juice and chicken broth

☐ **F.** Oatmeal and egg substitutes

ANSWER: C, D, E

Rationale: A clear liquid diet consists of foods that are clear liquids at room temperature or body temperature, such as ice pops, regular or decaffeinated coffee and tea, gelatin desserts, broth, carbonated beverages, and clear juices, such as apple and cranberry juices. Milk, pasteurized eggs, egg substitutes, and oatmeal are part of a full liquid diet.

Nursing process step: Implementation

Client needs category: Physiological integrity

Client needs subcategory: Basic care and comfort

Cognitive level: Comprehension

---

8. The nurse is teaching a pregnant client how to perform pelvic exercises to improve bladder control. What is the term for these exercises?

ANSWER: Kegel

Rationale: Kegel exercises are isometric exercises of the pelvic diaphragm muscles and perineum muscles that are used to improve vaginal contractility and bladder control.

Nursing process step: Implementation

Client needs category: Physiological integrity

Client needs subcategory: Basic care and comfort

Cognitive level: Application

9. The nurse is caring for a 16-year-old pregnant client who is taking an iron supplement. Which vitamin should the nurse instruct the client to take in order to increase iron absorption?

10. The nurse is palpating the uterus of a client who is 20 weeks pregnant in order to measure fundal height. Identify the area on the abdomen where the nurse should expect to feel the uterine fundus.

Answer:

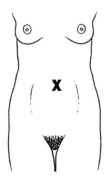

Rationale: At 20 weeks, fundal height should be at approximately the umbilicus. Fundal height should be measured from the symphysis pubis to the top of the uterus. Serial measurements assess fetal growth over the course of the pregnancy. Between weeks 18 and 34, the centimeters measured correlate approximately with the week of gestation.

Nursing process step: Data collection

Client needs category: Health promotion and maintenance

Client needs subcategory: Growth and development through the life span

Cognitive level: Comprehension

11. The nurse is teaching a course on the anatomy and physiology of reproduction. In the illustration of the female reproductive organs, identify the area where fertilization occurs.

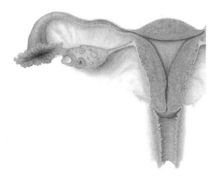

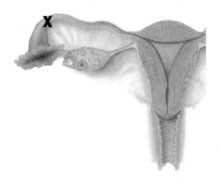

Rationale: After ejaculation, the sperm travel by flagellar movement through the fluids of the cervical mucus into the fallopian tube to meet the descending ovum in the ampulla. This is where fertilization occurs.

Nursing process step: Implementation

Client needs category: Health promotion and maintenance

Client needs subcategory: Growth and development through the life span

Cognitive level: Application

---

12. A client who is 14 weeks pregnant mentions she has been having difficulty moving her bowels since she became pregnant. What hormone is responsible for this common discomfort during pregnancy?

ANSWER: Progesterone

Rationale: Progesterone increases smooth muscle relaxation, thereby decreasing peristalsis. This slowed movement of contents through the GI system can lead to firmer stools and constipation.

Nursing process step: Data collection

Client needs category: Health promotion and maintenance

Client needs subcategory: Growth and development through the life span

Cognitive level: Application

13. In early pregnancy, some clients complain of abdominal pain or pulling. Identify the area most commonly associated with this pain.

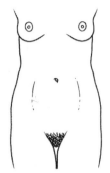

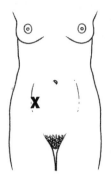

Rationale: As the uterus grows in early pregnancy, it deviates physically to the right. This shift, or dextrorotation, is due to the presence of the rectosigmoid colon in the left lower quadrant. As a result, many women complain of pain in the right lower quadrant.

Nursing process step: Evaluation

Client needs category: Health promotion and maintenance

Client needs subcategory: Growth and development through the life span

Cognitive level: Analysis

Intrapartum period

1. A client in the first stage of labor is being monitored using an external fetal monitor. The nurse notes variable decelerations on the monitoring strip. Into what position should the nurse assist the client?

Answer: Left lateral

Rationale: Variable decelerations are transient drops in fetal heart rate that occur before, during, or after a contraction. The left lateral position is the ideal position for any pregnant client because it prevents maternal hypotension caused by inferior vena cava compression, which reduces placental perfusion.

Nursing process step: Implementation

Client needs category: Physiological integrity

Client needs subcategory: Reduction of risk potential

Cognitive level: Analysis

2. A client with diabetes gives birth to a 9-lb, 10-oz neonate at 38 weeks. Which of the neonate's serum levels should be assessed immediately after birth?

_____

ANSWER: Glucose

Rationale: Glucose monitoring of the infant born to a mother with diabetes is essential because he is at risk for developing hypoglycemia after birth.

Nursing process step: Evaluation

Client needs category: Physiological integrity

Client needs subcategory: Reduction of risk potential

Cognitive level: Application

3. The nurse is assisting in monitoring a client who is receiving oxytocin (Pitocin) to induce labor. The nurse should be alert to which of the following maternal adverse reactions?

Select all that apply:

☑ **A.** Hypertension

☐ **B.** Jaundice

☐ **C.** Dehydration

☑ **D.** Fluid overload

☑ **E.** Uterine tetany

☐ **F.** Bradycardia

ANSWER: A, D, E

Rationale: Adverse effects of oxytocin in the mother include hypertension, fluid overload, and uterine tetany. Oxytocin's antidiuretic effect increases renal reabsorption of water, leading to fluid overload—not dehydration. Jaundice and bradycardia are adverse effects that may occur in the neonate. Tachycardia—not bradycardia—is reported as a maternal adverse effect.

Nursing process step: Planning

Client needs category: Physiological integrity

Client needs subcategory: Pharmacological therapies

Cognitive level: Application

4. The nurse is caring for a client who has been diagnosed with abruptio placentae. What signs and symptoms of abruptio placentae should the nurse expect to find when she is collecting data on this client?

Select all that apply:

☑ **A.** Vaginal bleeding

☐ **B.** Decreased fundal height

☑ **C.** Uterine tenderness on palpation

☐ **D.** Soft abdomen on palpation

☐ **E.** Hypotonic, small uterus

☑ **F.** Abnormal fetal heart tones

ANSWER: A, C, F

Rationale: Painful vaginal bleeding, uterine tenderness on palpation, and abnormal or absent heart tones are signs of abruptio placentae. Fundal height increases during abruptio placentae as a result of blood becoming trapped behind the placenta. The abdomen would feel hard and boardlike on palpation as blood permeates the myometrium and causes uterine irritability. The uterus would also be hypertonic and enlarged.

Nursing process step: Data collection

Client needs category: Physiological integrity

Client needs subcategory: Physiological adaptation

Cognitive level: Comprehension

---

5. The nurse is collecting data on a client in labor. She notes that the fetal heart rate is 110 beats/minute. What term describes this fetal heart rate?

ANSWER: Bradycardia

Rationale: A fetal heart rate of less than 120 beats/minute is known as fetal bradycardia.

Nursing process step: Data collection

Client needs category: Health promotion and maintenance

Client needs subcategory: Prevention and early detection of disease

Cognitive level: Knowledge

6. A nurse is assigned to assist with the admission of a client who is in labor. Which of the following actions are appropriate?

Select all that apply:

- ☑ **A.** Asking about the estimated date of delivery (EDD)
- ☐ **B.** Estimating fetal size
- ☑ **C.** Taking maternal and fetal vital signs
- ☐ **D.** Asking about the woman's last menses
- ☐ **E.** Administering an analgesic
- ☑ **F.** Asking about the amount of time between contractions

ANSWER: A, C, F

Rationale: The nurse should ask about the EDD and then compare the response to the information in the prenatal record. If the fetus is preterm, special precautions and equipment are necessary. Maternal and fetal vital signs should be obtained to evaluate the well-being of the client and fetus. Determining how far apart the contractions are provides the health care team with valuable baseline information. The physician estimates the size of the fetus. It wouldn't be appropriate for the nurse to ask about the client's last menses. This information should be collected at the first prenatal visit. It would be premature to administer an analgesic, which could slow or stop labor contractions.

Nursing process step: Implementation

Client needs category: Health promotion and maintenance

Client needs subcategory: Growth and development through the life span

Cognitive level: Application

---

7. The nurse is assisting in the delivery room. The physician makes an incision in the client's perineum to enlarge the vaginal opening and facilitate delivery. The nurse should document this as what procedure in the client's medical record?

_____

ANSWER: Episiotomy

Rationale: An episiotomy is surgical enlargement of the vaginal opening that allows easier delivery of the fetus. The incision, which is made in the perineum, can be midline, right, or left mediolateral.

Nursing process step: Implementation

Client needs category: Physiological integrity

Client needs subcategory: Reduction of risk potential

Cognitive level: Knowledge

8. The nurse is assisting in caring for a client who has just given birth to a neonate through vaginal delivery. The nurse is monitoring for signs of placental separation. Which of the following signs indicate that the placenta has separated?

Select all that apply:

☐ **A.** Shortening of the umbilical cord

☐ **B.** Sudden, sharp abdominal pain

☑ **C.** Sudden gush of vaginal blood

☑ **D.** Change in shape of the uterus

☑ **E.** Lengthening of the umbilical cord

ANSWER: C, D, E

Rationale: Signs of placental separation include lengthening of the umbilical cord, a sudden gush of blood from the vagina, a firmly contracted uterus, and change in uterine shape from discoid to globular. Sudden, sharp abdominal pain could indicate uterine rupture.

Nursing process step: Data collection

Client needs category: Physiological integrity

Client needs subcategory: Physiological adaptation

Cognitive level: Comprehension

---

9. A client in labor is 8 cm dilated. The fetus, which is in vertex presentation, is 75% effaced and is at 0 station. In the illustration below, identify the level of the fetus's head.

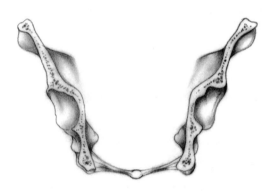

ANSWER:

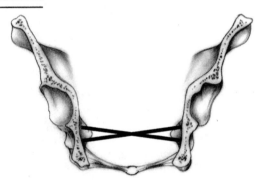

Rationale: Station refers to the level of the presenting part in relation to the pelvic inlet and the ischial spines. A 0 station indicates that the presenting part lies at the level of the ischial spines. Other stations are defined by their distance in centimeters above or below the ischial spines.

Nursing process step: Data collection

Client needs category: Health promotion and maintenance

Client needs subcategory: Growth and development through the life span

Cognitive level: Application

---

10. A primigravida experiences spontaneous rupture of the membranes. What rate should the nurse immediately check after the membranes rupture?

_____

ANSWER: Fetal heart rate

Rationale: When membranes rupture, the nurse should immediately check fetal heart rate to detect changes associated with prolapse or compression of the umbilical cord.

Nursing process step: Implementation

Client needs category: Physiological integrity

Client needs subcategory: Reduction of risk potential

Cognitive level: Application

Postpartum period

1. On examining a client who gave birth 3 hours ago, the nurse finds that the client has completely saturated a perineal pad within 15 minutes. Which of the following actions should the nurse take?

Select all that apply:

☐ **A.** Begin an I.V. infusion of lactated Ringer's solution.

☐ **B.** Assess the client's vital signs.

☐ **C.** Palpate the client's fundus.

☐ **D.** Place the client in high Fowler's position.

☐ **E.** Administer a pain medication.

ANSWER: B, C

Rationale: Assessing vital signs provides information about the client's circulatory status and identifies significant changes that may need to be reported to the physician. By palpating the client's fundus, the nurse also gains valuable assessment data. A boggy uterus may lead to excessive bleeding. Starting an I.V. infusion requires a physician's order. Placing the client in high Fowler's position may lower the blood pressure and be harmful to the client. Administration of a pain medication does not address the current problem.

Nursing process step: Data collection

Client needs category: Physiological integrity

Client needs subcategory: Reduction of risk potential

Cognitive level: Application

2. The nurse observes several interactions between a mother and her new son. Which of the following behaviors by the mother would the nurse identify as evidence of mother-infant attachment?

Select all that apply:

☑ **A.** Talks and coos to her son

☑ **B.** Cuddles her son close to her

☐ **C.** Doesn't make eye contact with her son

☐ **D.** Requests the nurse to take the baby to the nursery for feedings

☐ **E.** Encourages the father to hold the baby

☐ **F.** Takes a nap when the baby is sleeping

ANSWER: A, B

Rationale: Talking to, cooing to, and cuddling with her son are positive signs that the mother is adapting to her new role. Avoiding eye contact is a sign that the mother is not bonding with her baby. Eye contact, touching, and speaking are important to establish attachment with an infant. Feeding a neonate is an important role of a new mother and facilitates attachment. Encouraging the dad to hold the baby facilitates attachment between the newborn and the father. Resting while the infant is sleeping conserves needed energy and allows the mother to be alert and awake when her infant is awake; however, it isn't evidence of bonding.

Nursing process step: Evaluation

Client needs category: Psychosocial integrity

Client needs subcategory: Psychosocial adaptation

Cognitive level: Analysis

---

3. The nurse is instructing the client on breastfeeding. Which instructions should she include to help the mother prevent mastitis?

Select all that apply:

☐ **A.** Wash your nipples with soap and water.

☑ **B.** Change the breast pads frequently.

☑ **C.** Expose your nipples to air part of each day.

☑ **D.** Wash your hands before handling your breast and breast-feeding.

☐ **E.** Make sure that the baby grasps only the nipple.

☐ **F.** Release the baby's grasp on the nipple before removing him from the breast.

ANSWER: B, C, D, F

Rationale: Because mastitis is an infection commonly associated with a break in the skin surface of the nipple, measures to prevent cracked and fissured nipples help to prevent mastitis. Changing breast pads frequently and exposing the nipples to air part of the day help keep the nipples dry and prevent irritation. Washing the hands before handling the breast reduces the chance of accidentally introducing organisms into the breast. Releasing the baby's grasp on the nipple before removing the baby from the breast also reduces the chance of irritation. Nipples should be washed with water only. Soap can remove the body's natural oils and increases the chance of cracking. The baby should grasp both the nipple and areola.

Nursing process step: Planning

Client needs category: Health promotion and maintenance

Client needs subcategory: Prevention and early detection of disease

Cognitive level: Comprehension

4. The nurse is assessing the vaginal discharge of a client who is 1 day postpartum. The nurse notes that the discharge is dark red and contains shreds of decidua and mucus. What term should the nurse use in her nurse's notes to describe the discharge?

_____

ANSWER: Lochia rubra

Rationale: For the first 3 days after birth, lochia discharge consists almost entirely of blood with only small amounts of decidua and mucus. Because of its red color, it's called _lochia rubra_.

Nursing process step: Data collection

Client needs category: Physiological integrity

Client needs subcategory: Physiological adaptation

Cognitive level: Knowledge

5. The nurse is palpating a postpartum client's fundus. The client states, "I notice that my fundus is lower in my abdomen than yesterday." The nurse acknowledges this fact and explains that the client's uterus will progressively return to its prepregnancy state. She explains to the client that this process is known as what?

_____

ANSWER: Involution

Rationale: Involution is the progressive descent of the uterus into the pelvic cavity to its prepregnancy state. Descent occurs at approximately 1 cm per day. Clients who breast-feed may experience more rapid involution.

Nursing process step: Implementation

Client needs category: Health promotion and maintenance

Client needs subcategory: Prevention and early detection of disease

Cognitive level: Comprehension

6. The nurse is providing teaching to a postpartum client who has decided to breast-feed her neonate. The client wants to know how many extra calories she should eat. How many additional calories should the nurse instruct the client to eat per day?

_____

ANSWER: 500

Rationale: The recommended energy intake for a lactating mother is 500 kcal more than her prepregnancy intake.

Nursing process step: Implementation

Client needs category: Health promotion and maintenance

Client needs subcategory: Growth and development through the life span

Cognitive level: Application

---

7. In the fourth stage of labor, a full bladder increases the risk of which postpartum complication?

_____

ANSWER: Hemorrhage

Rationale: A full bladder prevents the uterus from contracting completely, increasing the risk of hemorrhage.

Nursing process step: Data collection

Client needs category: Physiological integrity

Client needs subcategory: Reduction of risk potential

Cognitive level: Knowledge

8. The nurse is palpating the uterine fundus of a client who delivered 8 hours ago. At what level in the abdomen would the nurse expect to feel the fundus?

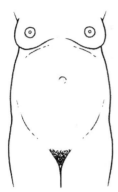

ANSWER:

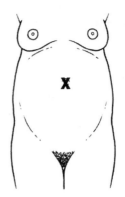

Rationale: The nurse should be able to feel the uterus at the level of the umbilicus from 1 hour after birth to approximately 24 hours after birth.

Nursing process step: Data collection

Client needs category: Physiological integrity

Client needs subcategory: Reduction of risk potential

Cognitive level: Comprehension

---

9. The nurse is assisting in developing a care plan for a client with an episiotomy. Which interventions would be included for the nursing diagnosis *Acute pain related to perineal sutures*?

Select all that apply:

☐ **A.** Apply an ice pack intermittently to the perineal area for 3 days.

☐ **B.** Avoid the use of topical pain gels.

☐ **C.** Administer sitz baths three to four times per day.

☐ **D.** Encourage the client to do Kegel exercises.

☐ **E.** Limit the number of times the perineal pad is changed.

ANSWER: C, D

Rationale: Sitz baths help decrease inflammation and tension in the perineal area. Kegel exercises improve circulation to the area and help reduce edema. Ice packs should be applied to the perineum for only the first 24 hours; after that time, heat should be used. Topical pain gels should be applied to the suture area to reduce discomfort, as ordered. The perineal pad should be changed frequently to prevent irritation caused by the discharge.

Nursing process step: Planning

Client needs category: Physiological integrity

Client needs subcategory: Basic care and comfort

Cognitive level: Application

1. The nurse is measuring the head circumference of a 1-hour-old neonate. She notices a raised bruised area on the left side of the head that does not cross the suture line. What is this called?

_____

ANSWER: Cephalhematoma

Rationale: A cephalhematoma is a collection of blood beneath the periosteum of the cranial bone that protrudes from the scalp. It may be seen on one or both sides of the head but does not cross the suture line. In comparison, caput succedaneum is a collection of fluid under the scalp that is bluish in color and may cross the suture line.

Nursing process step: Data collection

Client needs category: Physiological integrity

Client needs subcategory: Physiological adaptation

Cognitive level: Knowledge

---

2. A 14-day-old neonate is admitted for aspiration pneumonia. The results of a barium swallow confirm a diagnosis of gastroesophageal reflux with resulting aspiration pneumonia. Identify the area of the stomach that is weakened, contributing to the reflux.

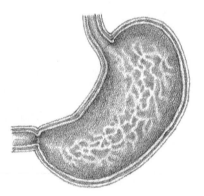

ANSWER:

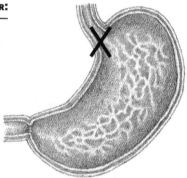

Rationale: Gastroesophageal reflux is a neuromotor disturbance in which the cardiac sphincter is lax and allows easy regurgitation of gastric contents into the esophagus, causing possible aspiration into the lungs. The cardiac sphincter is located between the stomach and the esophagus.

Nursing process step: Data collection

Client needs category: Physiological integrity

Client needs subcategory: Physiological adaptation

Cognitive level: Comprehension

3. In the nursery, the nurse is performing a neurologic assessment on a 1-day-old neonate. Which of the following findings would indicate possible asphyxia in utero?

Select all that apply:

☐ **A.** The neonate grasps the nurse's finger when she puts it in the palm of his hand.

☐ **B.** The neonate does stepping movements when held upright with his sole touching a surface.

☑ **C.** The neonate's toes don't curl downward when his soles are stroked.

☑ **D.** The neonate doesn't respond when the nurse claps her hands above him.

☐ **E.** The neonate turns toward an object when the nurse touches his cheek with it.

☐ **F.** The neonate displays weak, ineffective sucking.

ANSWER: C, D, F

Rationale: Failure of the toes to curl downward when the soles are stroked and lack of response to a loud sound can be evidence that neurological damage from asphyxia has occurred. The normal responses would be that the toes curl downward with stroking and the arms and legs extend in response to a loud noise. Weak, ineffective sucking is another sign of neurologic damage; a neonate should root and suck when the side of his cheek is stroked. A neonate should also grasp a person's finger when it is placed in the palm of his hand, do stepping movements when held upright with the soles touching a surface, and turn toward an object when his cheek is touched.

Nursing process step: Data collection

Client needs category: Health promotion and maintenance

Client needs subcategory: Growth and development through the life span

Cognitive level: Application

---

4. Which of the following instructions should the nurse provide on discharge from the facility to the parents of a neonate who has been circumcised?

Select all that apply:

☑ **A.** The infant must void before being discharged home.

☑ **B.** Apply petroleum jelly to the glans of the penis with each diaper change.

☐ **C.** Tub baths for the infant are acceptable while the circumcision heals.

☐ **D.** Report any blood on the front of the diaper.

☑ **E.** The circumcision requires care for 2 to 4 days after discharge.

ANSWER: A, B, E

Rationale: It's necessary for a circumcised infant to void prior to discharge to ensure that the urethra is not obstructed. A lubricating ointment, such as petroleum jelly, should be applied to the glans with each diaper change. Typically, the penis heals within 2 to 4 days and circumcision care is needed only during that period. Parents should avoid giving the neonate tub baths until the circumcision heals to prevent infection; only sponge baths are appropriate. A small amount of bleeding is expected after circumcision; parents should report only large amounts of bleeding to the physician.

Nursing process step: Implementation

Client needs category: Safe, effective care environment

Client needs subcategory: Coordinated care

Cognitive level: Application

5. The nurse is planning to administer an injection to a neonate that will help prevent abnormal bleeding. What vitamin is the nurse planning to administer?

_____

ANSWER: Vitamin K

Rationale: Vitamin K is necessary for the body to synthesize coagulation factors, which help to prevent abnormal bleeding. A neonate is deficient in vitamin K because his bowel doesn't have the bacteria necessary for synthesizing it.

Nursing process step: Implementation

Client needs category: Physiological integrity

Client needs subcategory: Pharmacological therapies

Cognitive level: Application

---

6. The nurse is eliciting reflexes in a neonate during a physical examination. Identify the area the nurse would touch to elicit a plantar grasp reflex.

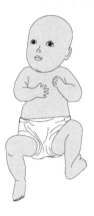

ANSWER:

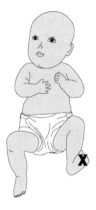

Rationale: Touching the sole of the foot near the base of the digits elicits a plantar grasp reflex and causes flexion or grasping. This reflex disappears around age 9 months.

Nursing process step: Data collection

Client needs category: Health promotion and maintenance

Client needs subcategory: Growth and development through the life span

Cognitive level: Application

7. The nurse notes that at 5 minutes after birth, a neonate is pink with acrocyanosis, has his knees flexed and fists clinched, has a whimpering cry, has a heart rate of 128 beats/minute, and withdraws his foot to a slap on the sole. What 5-minute Apgar score should the nurse record for this neonate?

Sign	Apgar Score		
	0	1	2
Heart rate	Absent	Less than 100 beats/minute (slow)	More than 100 beats/minute
Respirator effort	Absent	Slow, irregular	Good crying
Muscle tone	Flaccid	Some flexion and resistance to extension of extremities	Active motion
Reflex irritability	No response	Grimace or weak cry	Vigorous cry
Color	Pallor, cyanosis	Pink body, blue extremities	Completely pink

Rationale: The Apgar score quantifies neonatal heart rate, respiratory effort, muscle tone, reflexes, and color. Each category is assessed 1 minute after birth and again 5 minutes later. Scores in each category range from 0 to 2, as shown below. This neonate has a heart rate above 100 beats/minute, which equals 2; is pink in color with acrocyanosis, which equals 1; is well-flexed, which equals 2; has a weak cry, which equals 1; and has a good response to slapping the soles, which equals 2. Therefore, the nurse should record a total Apgar score of 8.

Nursing process step: Data collection

Client needs category: Physiological integrity

Client needs subcategory: Physiological adaptation

Cognitive level: Analysis

---

8. The nurse is demonstrating cord care to a mother of a neonate. Which actions should the nurse teach the mother to perform?

Select all that apply:

☑ **A.** Explain that the diaper is kept below the cord.

☐ **B.** Tug gently on the cord to remove it as it begins to dry.

☐ **C.** Apply antibiotic ointment to the cord twice daily.

☑ **D.** Only sponge-bathe the infant until the cord falls off.

☑ **E.** Clean the length of the cord with alcohol several times daily.

☐ **F.** Wash the cord with mild soap and water.

Rationale: The diaper should be positioned below the cord to allow for it to air dry and to prevent urine from getting on it. Parents should be instructed to sponge-bathe the infant until the cord falls off; soap and water should not be used. The entire cord should be cleaned with alcohol, using a cotton-tipped applicator or another appropriate method. Parents should also be instructed to never pull on the cord; they should allow it to fall off naturally. Antibiotic ointments are contraindicated unless signs of infection are present.

Nursing process step: Planning

Client needs category: Safe, effective care environment

Client needs subcategory: Safety and infection control

Cognitive level: Application

Part 4
Pediatric nursing

1. The physician orders digoxin 0.1 mg orally every morning for a 6-month-old infant with heart failure. Digoxin is available in a 400 mcg/ml concentration. How many milliliters of digoxin should the nurse give?

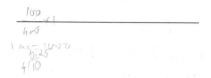

Answer: 0.25

Rationale:

To convert mg to mcg:

$$1{,}000 \text{ mcg}/1 \text{ mg} = X \text{ mcg}/0.1 \text{ mg}$$

$$X = 100 \text{ mcg}$$

To calculate drug dose:

Dose on hand/Quantity on hand = Dose desired/X

$$400 \text{ mcg/ml} = 100 \text{ mcg}/X$$

$$X = 0.25 \text{ ml}$$

Nursing process step: Implementation

Client needs category: Physiological integrity

Client needs subcategory: Pharmacological therapies

Cognitive level: Application

---

2. What muscle is the primary site for intramuscular injections in infants?

Answer: Vastus lateralis

Rationale: The vastus lateralis is the preferred site for intramuscular injections in infants because it doesn't have major nerve endings and blood vessels. The ventrogluteal site may only be used if the child has been walking for 1 year. The dorsogluteal site has a high risk for sciatic nerve damage and is poorly developed in infants. The deltoid muscle site has a small muscle mass, which limits the amount of medication that can be injected into it at one time.

Nursing process step: Planning

Client needs category: Physiological integrity

Client needs subcategory: Pharmacological therapies

Cognitive level: Application

3. According to Erickson, what is the psychosocial stage of development for an infant?

_____

ANSWER: Trust versus mistrust

Rationale: Erickson labels an infant's psychosocial stage of development as a stage of trust versus mistrust. The quality of the caregiver-infant relationship and the consistency of care help the infant develop trust. When care is inconsistent and the infant experiences a delay in gratification of needs, uncertainty and mistrust can develop.

Nursing process step: Data collection

Client needs category: Health promotion and maintenance

Client needs subcategory: Growth and development through the life span

Cognitive level: Comprehension

---

4. The nurse is preparing to administer chloramphenicol (Chloromycetin Otic) to a 2-year-old with an infection of the external auditory canal. The order reads, "2 gtts A.D. t.i.d." Which steps should the nurse take to administer this medication?

Select all that apply:

☑ **A.** Wash her hands and arrange supplies at the bedside.

☐ **B.** Warm the medication to body temperature.

☐ **C.** Lie the child on his right side with his left ear facing up.

☐ **D.** Examine the ear canal for drainage.

☐ **E.** Gently pull the pinna up and back and instill the drops into the external ear canal.

ANSWER: A, B, D

Rationale: The nurse should prepare to instill the eardrops by washing her hands, gathering the supplies, and arranging the supplies at the bedside. To avoid adverse effects resulting from eardrops that are too cold (such as vertigo, nausea, and pain), the medication should be warmed to body temperature in a bowl of warm water. Temperature of the drops should be tested by placing a drop on the wrist. Before instilling the drops, the ear canal should be examined for drainage that may reduce the medication's effectiveness. Because the abbreviation "A.D." stands for "right ear," the child should be placed on his left side with his right ear facing up. For an infant or a child younger than age 3, gently pull the auricle down and back because the ear canal is straighter in children of this age-group.

Nursing process step: Implementation

Client needs category: Physiological integrity

Client needs subcategory: Pharmacological therapies

Cognitive level: Application

5. The nurse is caring for a 1-month-old infant who fell from the changing table during a diaper change. Which signs and symptoms of increased intracranial pressure (ICP) is the nurse likely to assess in a 1-month-old infant?

Select all that apply:

☐ **A.** Bulging fontanels

☐ **B.** Decreased blood pressure

☐ **C.** Increased pulse

☑ **D.** High-pitched cry

☐ **E.** Headache

☑ **F.** Irritability

ANSWER: A, D, F

Rationale: Signs and symptoms of increased ICP in a 1-month-old include full, tense, bulging fontanels; a high-pitched cry; and irritability. With increased ICP, blood pressure rises while heart rate falls. The infant may have a headache, but the nurse is unable to assess this finding in an infant.

Nursing process step: Data collection

Client needs category: Physiological integrity

Client needs subcategory: Physiological adaptation

Cognitive level: Analysis

---

6. An 11-month-old is diagnosed with an ear infection, his second one. The mother asks why children experience more ear infections than adults. The nurse shows the mother a diagram of the ear and explains the differences in anatomy. Identify the portion of the infant's ear that allows fluid to stagnate and act as a medium for bacteria.

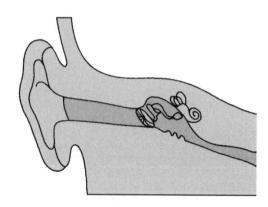

ANSWER:

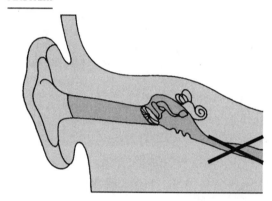

Rationale: The eustachian tube in an infant is shorter and wider than in an adult or an older child. It also slants horizontally. Because of these anatomical features, nasopharyngeal secretions can enter the middle ear more easily, stagnate, and tend to cause infections.

Nursing process step: Implementation

Client needs category: Health promotion and maintenance

Client needs subcategory: Growth and development through the life span

Cognitive level: Comprehension

7. The nurse is assessing a 10-month-old infant during a checkup. Which developmental milestones would the nurse expect the infant to display?

Select all that apply:

☐ **A.** Holding head erect

☐ **B.** Self-feeding

☐ **C.** Demonstrating good bowel and bladder control

☐ **D.** Sitting on a firm surface without support

☑ **E.** Bearing majority of weight on legs

☐ **F.** Walking alone

ANSWER: A, D, E

Rationale: By age 3 months, an infant should be able to hold his head erect. By age 10 months, he should be able to sit on a firm surface without support and bear the majority of his weight on his legs (for example, walking while holding on to furniture). Self-feeding and bowel and bladder control are developmental milestones of toddlers. By age 12 months, the infant should be able to stand alone and may take his first steps.

Nursing process step: Data collection

Client needs category: Health promotion and maintenance

Client needs subcategory: Growth and development through the life span

Cognitive level: Application

---

8. The nurse is teaching cardiopulmonary resuscitation (CPR) to the parents of a 1-month-old being discharged with an apnea monitor. Which steps are appropriate for performing CPR on an infant?

Select all that apply:

☐ **A.** Open the airway by hyperextending the head.

☐ **B.** Pinch the nose before delivering a breath.

☑ **C.** Check for a pulse by palpating the brachial artery.

☐ **D.** Place the heel of one hand on the lower third of the sternum to perform compressions.

☑ **E.** Compress the sternum ½″ to 1″.

☑ **F.** Give five compressions to one breath.

ANSWER: C, E, F

Rationale: When performing CPR on an infant, check for a brachial pulse by palpating the inside of the upper arm, midway between the elbow and shoulder. To provide compressions to an infant, compress the sternum ½″ to 1″ at a ratio of five compressions to one breath. Tilting the head too far back in an infant can block, rather than open, the airway. To deliver a breath to an infant, the rescuer should cover the infant's mouth and nose with her mouth. When performing chest compressions on an infant, the tips of the middle and ring fingers should be placed on the sternum, one finger's width below the nipple line.

Nursing process step: Implementation

Client needs category: Physiological integrity

Client needs subcategory: Reduction of risk potential

Cognitive level: Application

9. The nurse is providing preoperative teaching to the parents of a 9-month-old infant who is having surgery to repair a ventricular septal defect. Identify the area of the heart where the defect is located.

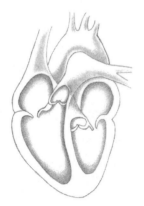

ANSWER:

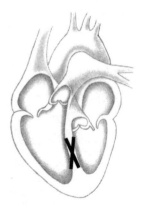

Rationale: A ventricular septal defect is a hole in the septum between the ventricles. The defect can be anywhere along the septum but is most commonly located in the middle of the septum.

Nursing process step: Implementation

Client needs category: Physiological integrity

Client needs subcategory: Physiological adaptation

Cognitive level: Comprehension

---

10. A nurse at the family clinic receives a call from the mother of a 5-week-old infant. The mother states that her child was diagnosed with colic at the last checkup. Unfortunately, the symptoms have remained the same. Which teaching instructions are appropriate?

Select all that apply:

☐ **A.** Position the infant on his back after feedings.

☐ **B.** Soothe the child by humming and rocking.

☐ **C.** Immediately bring the infant to the emergency department.

☐ **D.** Burp the infant adequately after feedings.

☐ **E.** Provide small but frequent feedings to the infant.

☐ **F.** Offer a pacifier if it isn't time for the infant to eat.

ANSWER: B, D, E, F

Rationale: Colic consists of recurrent paroxysmal bouts of abdominal pain and is fairly common in infants. It usually disappears by age 3 months. Rocking, riding in a car, humming, and offering a pacifier may be used to comfort the infant. Decreasing gas formation by frequent burping, giving smaller feedings more frequently, and positioning the infant in an upright seat are also appropriate teaching. The infant shouldn't be positioned on his back after feedings because this increases gas formation. Colic is a manageable condition in the home. The infant doesn't need to be taken to the emergency department unless the symptoms worsen, a temperature accompanies the symptoms, or vomiting occurs with the symptoms.

Nursing process step: Implementation

Client needs category: Physiological integrity

Client needs subcategory: Basic care and comfort

Cognitive level: Application

11.

A 6-month-old is found floating face down in a swimming pool. A neighbor, who is a nurse, assesses for the presence of respirations and a pulse. Identify the area that is most appropriate to check for a pulse.

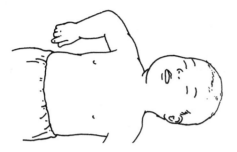

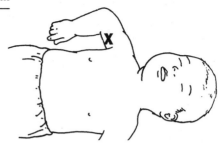

Rationale: An infant's pulse is most accessible at the brachial artery. The brachial artery is located inside the upper arm between the elbow and the shoulder. Cardiopulmonary resuscitation guidelines recommend using this area to assess for a pulse.

Nursing process step: Implementation

Client needs category: Physiological integrity

Client needs subcategory: Physiological adaptation

Cognitive level: Application

---

12. The nurse is teaching the parents of an infant undergoing repair for a cleft lip. Which instructions should the nurse give?

Select all that apply:

- ☐ **A.** Offer a pacifier as needed.
- ☐ **B.** Lay the infant on his back or side to sleep.
- ☐ **C.** Sit the infant up for each feeding.
- ☐ **D.** Loosen the arm restraints every 4 hours.
- ☐ **E.** Clean the suture line after each feeding by dabbing it with saline solution.
- ☐ **F.** Give the infant extra care and support.

ANSWER: B, C, E, F

Rationale: An infant with a repaired cleft lip should be put to sleep on his back or side to prevent trauma to the surgery site. He should be fed in the upright position with a syringe and attached tubing to prevent stress to the suture line from sucking. To prevent crusts and scarring, the suture line should be cleaned after each feeding by dabbing it with half-strength hydrogen peroxide or saline solution. The infant should receive extra care and support because he can't meet emotional needs by sucking. Extra care and support may also prevent crying, which stresses the suture line. Pacifiers shouldn't be used during the healing process because they stress the suture line. Arm restraints are used to keep the infant's hands away from the mouth and should be loosened every 2 hours.

Nursing process step: Implementation

Client needs category: Physiological integrity

Client needs subcategory: Reduction of risk potential

Cognitive level: Application

1. The nurse is admitting a 14-month-old to the pediatric floor with diagnosis of croup. Which characteristics would the nurse expect the toddler to have if he is developing normally?

Select all that apply:

☐ **A.** Strong hand grasp

☐ **B.** Tendency to hold one object while looking for another

☐ **C.** Recognition of familiar voices (smiles in recognition)

☐ **D.** Presence of Moro reflex

☐ **E.** Weight that is triple the birth weight

☐ **F.** Closed anterior fontanelle

ANSWER: A, B, C, AND E

Rationale: A strong hand grasp is demonstrated within the first month of life. Holding one object while looking for another is accomplished by the 20th week. Within the first year of life, the toddler masters smiling at familiar faces and voices, the Moro reflex disappears, and birth weight triples. The anterior fontanel closes at approximately age 18 months.

Nursing process step: Data collection

Client needs category: Health promotion and maintenance

Client needs subcategory: Growth and development through the life span

Cognitive level: Application

---

2. A 13-month-old is admitted to the pediatric unit with a diagnosis of gastroenteritis. The toddler has experienced vomiting and diarrhea for the past 3 days, and laboratory tests reveal that he is dehydrated. Which nursing interventions are correct to prevent further dehydration?

Select all that apply:

☐ **A.** Encourage the child to eat a balanced diet.

☐ **B.** Give clear liquids in small amounts.

☐ **C.** Give milk in small amounts.

☐ **D.** Encourage the child to eat nonsalty soups and broths.

☐ **E.** Monitor the I.V. solution per the physician's order.

☐ **F.** Withhold all solid food and liquids until the symptoms pass.

ANSWER: B, D, E

Rationale: A child experiencing nausea and vomiting would not be able to tolerate a regular diet. He should be given sips of clear liquids, and the diet should be advanced as tolerated. Unsalty soups and broths are appropriate clear liquids. Milk should not be given because it can worsen the child's diarrhea. I.V. fluids should be monitored to maintain the fluid status and help to rehydrate the child. Solid foods may be withheld throughout the acute phase; however, clear fluids should be encouraged in small amounts (3 to 4 tablespoons every half hour).

Nursing process step: Implementation

Client needs category: Physiological integrity

Client needs subcategory: Basic care and comfort

Cognitive level: Application

---

3. An acutely ill, 20-month-old toddler is admitted to the hospital with a vaso-occlusive sickle cell crisis. The child is crying and restless and appears uncomfortable when touched. What nursing diagnosis would the nurse expect to be included in the care plan?

_____

ANSWER: Acute pain

Rationale: In a vaso-occlusive crisis, sickle-shaped cells stick and clump together, obstructing normal blood flow. A thrombus may form and obstruct circulation, possibly leading to tissue death. Severe pain in the affected body parts is the characteristic symptom when tissue is denied normal blood circulation.

Nursing process step: Planning

Client needs category: Physiological integrity

Client needs subcategory: Basic care and comfort

Cognitive level: Comprehension

---

4. A toddler is ordered 350 mg of amoxicillin (Augmentin) by mouth, four times per day. The pharmacy sends a bottle of amoxicillin with a concentration of 250 mg/5 ml. How many milliliters should the nurse administer per dose?

_____

ANSWER: 7

Rationale: The following formula is used to calculate drug dosages: Dose on hand/Quantity on hand = Dose desired/X. In this example, the equation is 250 mg/5 ml = 350 mg/X. X = 7 ml.

Nursing process step: Implementation

Client needs category: Physiological integrity

Client needs subcategory: Pharmacological therapies

Cognitive level: Application

5. A 3-year-old is admitted to the pediatric unit with pneumonia. He has a productive cough and appears to have difficulty breathing. The parents tell the nurse that the toddler hasn't been eating or drinking much and has been very inactive. Which interventions to improve airway clearance should the nurse include in the care plan?

Select all that apply:

☐ **A.** Restrict fluid intake.

☑ **B.** Perform chest physiotherapy as ordered.

☑ **C.** Encourage coughing and deep breathing.

☐ **D.** Keep the head of the bed flat.

☑ **E.** Perform postural drainage.

☑ **F.** Maintain humidification with a cool mist humidifier.

ANSWER: B, C, E, F

Rationale: Chest physiotherapy and postural drainage work together to break up congestion and then drain secretions. Coughing and deep breathing are also effective to remove congestion. A cool mist humidifier helps loosen thick mucus and relax airway passages. Fluids should be encouraged — not restricted. The child should be placed in semi-Fowler's or high Fowler's position to facilitate breathing and promote optimal lung expansion.

Nursing process step: Implementation

Client needs category: Physiological integrity

Client needs subcategory: Basic care and comfort

Cognitive level: Application

The preschooler

1. The nurse is observing the parents of a 4-year-old who has been admitted to the hospital. Which of the following actions indicate that the parents understand how to best minimize anxiety during their child's hospitalization?

Select all that apply:

☑ **A.** The parents bring the child's favorite toy to the hospital.

☐ **B.** The parents explain all procedures to the child in great detail.

☑ **C.** The parents remain at the child's side during the hospitalization.

☑ **D.** The parents bring the child's siblings for a brief visit.

☐ **E.** The parents leave the room when the child undergoes a painful procedure.

☐ **F.** The parents punish the child if the child isn't cooperative.

ANSWER: A, C, D

Rationale: The most effective means of minimizing the child's anxiety during hospitalization is to have the parents stay with him. Having a familiar toy helps the child to deal with the anxiety of unfamiliar surroundings. Sibling visitation can also help to ease the child's anxiety. Explaining a procedure to a young child in great detail only maximizes fear. Parents can be effective in calming and comforting a child during painful procedures, so they should remain in the room. Rewards, not punishment, should be offered to a preschooler.

Nursing process step: Evaluation

Client needs category: Psychosocial integrity

Client needs subcategory: Coping and adaptation

Cognitive level: Analysis

2. A 5-year-old suspected of having leukemia is admitted to the hospital for diagnosis and treatment. Which test should the nurse most expect to be performed to confirm the diagnosis of leukemia?

_____

ANSWER: Bone marrow aspiration

Rationale: Bone marrow aspiration and analysis are necessary to confirm the diagnosis of leukemia. The bone marrow of a child with leukemia is characterized by hypercellularity, lack of fat globules, and presence of blast cells (immature white cells).

Nursing process step: Planning

Client needs category: Physiological integrity

Client needs subcategory: Physiological adaptation

Cognitive level: Knowledge

3. Which category of transmission precautions is most appropriate for the hospitalized preschooler who has varicella (chickenpox)?

_____

ANSWER: Airborne

Rationale: Airborne precautions are appropriate because varicella is transmitted by airborne droplet nuclei.

Nursing process step: Implementation

Client needs category: Safe, effective care environment

Client needs subcategory: Safety and infection control

Cognitive level: Knowledge

4. A 5-year-old is admitted to the hospital for a tonsillectomy. After the surgery, the physician orders a clear liquid diet. The nurse is correct in giving the child which of the following items?

Select all that apply:

☐ **A.** Cream of chicken soup

☐ **B.** Orange juice

☐ **C.** Ice cream

☐ **D.** Apple juice

☐ **E.** Lime gelatin

☐ **F.** Chicken broth

ANSWER: D, E, F

Rationale: Clear liquids include clear broth, gelatin, clear juices, water, and ice chips. Cream of chicken soup, orange juice, and ice cream are included in a full liquid diet.

Nursing process step: Implementation

Client needs category: Physiological integrity

Client needs subcategory: Basic care and comfort

Cognitive level: Application

---

5. A 5-year-old is brought to the emergency department with a fever, severe vomiting, irritability, and confusion. The parents state that the child had a recent viral illness but was recovering without difficulty. Numerous diagnostic studies are completed, yielding the results of acute encephalopathy as well as fatty degeneration of the liver and other abdominal organs. Reye's syndrome is diagnosed. Which medication should the nurse suspect was given to the child during his illness?

ANSWER: Aspirin

Rationale: Administration of aspirin during a viral illness has been implicated as a contributing factor in the development of Reye's syndrome.

Nursing process step: Data collection

Client needs category: Physiological integrity

Client needs subcategory: Pharmacological therapies

Cognitive level: Analysis

6. The school nurse is conducting registration for a first grader. Which of the following immunizations should the school nurse verify the child has had on entering school?

Select all that apply:

☑ **A.** Hepatitis B series

☑ **B.** Diphtheria-tetanus-pertussis series

☑ **C.** *Haemophilus influenzae* type b series

☐ **D.** Varicella zoster

☐ **E.** Pneumonia vaccine

☑ **F.** Oral polio series

ANSWER: A, B, C, F

Rationale: Hepatitis B series, diphtheria-tetanus-pertussis series, *H. influenzae* type b series, and oral polio series are immunizations that the child should receive before entering first grade. The varicella zoster vaccine is administered only if the child hasn't had chickenpox. Pneumonia vaccine isn't required or routinely given to children.

Nursing process step: Data collection

Client needs category: Health promotion and maintenance

Client needs subcategory: Prevention and early detection of disease

Cognitive level: Knowledge

---

7. A preschooler is in danger of becoming dehydrated as a result of vomiting and diarrhea. The nurse realizes that dehydration can be prevented if intake is sufficient to produce a urine output of 3 ml/kg/hr. The preschooler weighs 44 lb. What is the minimum urine output in milliliters that should be achieved in an 8-hour shift in order to prevent dehydration?

ANSWER: 480

Rationale: First, convert the child's weight from pounds to kilograms. There are 2.2 kg in 1 lb. Thus, 44 divided by 2.2 = 20, and 3 ml X 20 kg X 8 hours = 480.

Nursing process step: Planning

Client needs category: Physiological integrity

Client needs subcategory: Reduction of risk potential

Cognitive level: Comprehension

8. A preschooler is diagnosed with Wilms' tumor. In which structure of the urinary system is the tumor located?

Answer: Kidney

Rationale: Wilms' tumor, also called *nephroblastoma,* is located in the kidney. It most commonly occurs in children ages 2 to 4.

Nursing process step: Data collection

Client needs category: Physiological integrity

Client needs subcategory: Physiological adaptation

Cognitive level: Knowledge

The school-age child

1. The nurse in a pediatrician's office is assessing the cognitive ability of a 7-year-old child who is in first grade. The nurse places six blocks on the table and asks the child to count the blocks. The nurse then rearranges the blocks and asks the child for the total number of blocks. The child demonstrates an understanding of conservation of mass. According to Piaget, which developmental stage is the child exhibiting?

Answer: Concrete operational

Rationale: During the school-age years, the child's cognitive skills develop. At about age 7, children develop the ability to understand that a change in shape doesn't mean a change in mass or amount. Piaget defines this stage as the concrete operational stage.

Nursing process step: Evaluation

Client needs category: Health promotion and maintenance

Client needs subcategory: Growth and development through the life span

Cognitive level: Analysis

2. A 12-year-old is brought to the emergency department after a soccer game. The child complains of having difficulty breathing. When auscultating the child's lungs, the nurse hears the sound of expired air being pushed through obstructed bronchioles. What term should the nurse use to document this finding?

_____

Answer: Wheezes

Rationale: Wheezes are high-pitched sounds of expired air being pushed through a narrow airway.

Nursing process step: Data collection

Client needs category: Physiological integrity

Client needs subcategory: Physiological adaptation

Cognitive level: Comprehension

3. A 12-year-old boy with diabetes tests his glucose level before lunch at school using a glucometer. He receives a reading of 245 mg/dl and goes to see the school nurse. The nurse is most correct in using the ordered sliding scale for insulin coverage and administering which type of insulin for this glucometer reading?

_____

Answer: Regular

Rationale: Regular insulin is short-acting insulin that's used for sliding scale insulin coverage when the glucose level is elevated. Short-acting insulin has an onset of ½ hour to 1 hour.

Nursing process step: Implementation

Client needs category: Physiological integrity

Client needs subcategory: Pharmacological therapies

Cognitive level: Application

4. An 11-year-old boy is brought to a rural clinic listless and pale. The parents state that the child had a "bad sore throat" 2 weeks ago and that they had him gargle with salt water. The parents report that they saw improvement but now the child has flulike symptoms. The child is diagnosed with rheumatic fever. Which of the following signs and symptoms are associated with rheumatic fever?

Select all that apply:

☐ **A.** Nausea and vomiting

☐ **B.** Polyarthritis

☐ **C.** Chorea

☐ **D.** High-grade fever

☐ **E.** Carditis

☐ **F.** Rash

ANSWER: B, C, E, F

Rationale: Characteristic manifestations of rheumatic fever include polyarthritis, chorea, carditis, and a red rash. The child doesn't usually experience nausea and vomiting. He may have a minor low-grade fever in the afternoon.

Nursing process step: Implementation

Client needs category: Physiological integrity

Client needs subcategory: Physiological adaptation

Cognitive level: Application

---

5. When talking with 10- and 11-year-old children about death, the nurse should incorporate which guidelines?

Select all that apply:

☐ **A.** Logical explanations aren't appropriate.

☐ **B.** The children will be curious about the physical aspects of death.

☐ **C.** The children will know that death is inevitable and irreversible.

☐ **D.** The children will be influenced by the attitudes of the adults in their lives.

☐ **E.** Teaching about death and dying shouldn't start before age 11.

☐ **F.** Telling children that death is the same as going to sleep as a way of relieving fear is appropriate.

ANSWER: B, C, D

Rationale: By age 9 or 10, most children know that death is universal, inevitable, and irreversible. School-age children are curious about the physical aspects of death and may wonder what happens to the body. Their cognitive abilities are advanced and they respond well to logical explanations. They should be encouraged to ask questions. The adults in their environment influence their attitudes towards death. Adults should be encouraged to include children in the family rituals and should be prepared to answer questions that might seem shocking. Teaching about death should begin early in childhood. Comparing death to sleep can be frightening for children and cause them to fear falling asleep.

Nursing process step: Implementation

Client needs category: Psychosocial integrity

Client needs subcategory: Coping and adaptation

Cognitive level: Application

6. A 7-year-old client is admitted to the hospital for treatment of facial cellulitis. He is admitted for observation and for administration of a 10-day course of I.V. antibiotics. Which interventions would help this client cope with the insertion of a peripheral I.V. line?

Select all that apply:

☐ **A.** Explain the procedure to the child immediately before the procedure.

☐ **B.** Apply a topical anesthetic to the I.V. site before the procedure.

☐ **C.** Ask the child which hand he uses for drawing.

☐ **D.** Explain the procedure to the child using abstract terms.

☐ **E.** Don't let the child see the equipment to be used in the procedure.

☐ **F.** Tell the child that the procedure won't hurt.

ANSWER: B, C

Rationale: Topical anesthetics reduce the pain of a venipuncture. The cream should be applied about 1 hour before the procedure and requires a physician's order. Asking which hand the child draws with helps to identify the dominant hand. The I.V. should be inserted into the opposite extremity so that the child can continue to play and to do homework with a minimum amount of disruption. Younger school-age children don't have the capability for abstract thinking. The procedure should be explained using simple words. Definitions of unfamiliar terms should be provided. The child should have the procedure explained to him well before it takes place so that he has time to ask questions. Although the topical anesthetic will relieve some pain, there is usually some pain or discomfort involved in venipuncture, so the child shouldn't be told otherwise.

Nursing process step: Implementation

Client needs category: Psychosocial integrity

Client needs subcategory: Coping and adaptation

Cognitive level: Application

---

7. When teaching bicycle safety to children and parents, the nurse should stress using what protective equipment as a priority?

ANSWER: Helmet

Rationale: Head injury is the primary cause of bicycle-related fatalities in children. A well-fitting helmet is the safety feature that's most important to stress to children and parents.

Nursing process step: Implementation

Client needs category: Physiological integrity

Client needs subcategory: Reduction of risk potential

Cognitive level: Application

8. A 6-year-old female is brought to the pediatrician's office by her mother for evaluation. The child recently started wetting the bed and running a low-grade fever. A urinalysis is positive for bacteria and protein. A diagnosis of a urinary tract infection (UTI) is made and the child is prescribed antibiotics. Which interventions are appropriate?

Select all that apply:

☐ **A.** Limit fluids for the next few days to decrease the frequency of urination.

☐ **B.** Assess the mother's understanding of UTIs and its causes.

☐ **C.** Instruct the mother to administer the antibiotic as prescribed—even if the symptoms diminish.

☐ **D.** Provide instructions only to the mother, not the child.

☐ **E.** Discourage the use of bubble bath.

☐ **F.** Tell the mother to have the child wipe from the back to the front after voiding and defecation.

ANSWER: B, C, E

Rationale: Assessing the mother's understanding of UTI and its causes provides the nurse with a baseline for teaching. The full course of antibiotics must be given to eradicate the organism and prevent recurrence, even if the child's signs and symptoms decrease. Bubble bath can irritate the vulva and urethra and contribute to the development of a UTI. Fluids should be encouraged, not limited, in order to prevent urinary stasis and help flush the organism out of the urinary tract. Instructions should be given to the child at her level of understanding to help her better understand the treatment and promote compliance. The child should wipe from the front to the back, not back to front, to minimize the risk of contamination after elimination.

Nursing process step: Implementation

Client needs category: Health promotion and maintenance

Client needs subcategory: Prevention and early detection of disease

Cognitive level: Application

The adolescent

1. Which symptoms reported by an adolescent's parents indicate that the adolescent is abusing amphetamines?

Select all that apply:

☐ **A.** Restlessness

☐ **B.** Fatigue

☐ **C.** Excessive perspiration

☐ **D.** Talkativeness

☐ **E.** Watery eyes

☐ **F.** Excessive nasal drainage

ANSWER: A, C, D

Rationale: Amphetamines are central nervous system stimulants. Symptoms of amphetamine abuse include marked nervousness, restlessness, excitability, talkativeness, and excessive perspiration.

Nursing process step: Data collection

Client needs category: Health promotion and maintenance

Client needs subcategory: Prevention and early detection of disease

Cognitive level: Application

2. A group of 16-year-olds are eating at a restaurant. One adolescent starts to cough. He puts his hands around his neck to gesture that he can't breathe. A friend stands and positions himself to begin the Heimlich maneuver. Identify the area where it's most appropriate to place the hands when performing the Heimlich maneuver.

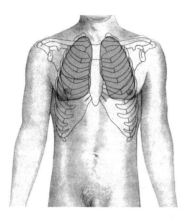

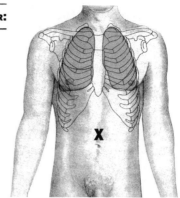

Rationale: To perform the Heimlich maneuver, the rescuer should place his hands on the abdomen, just above the navel.

Nursing process step: Implementation

Client needs category: Physiological integrity

Client needs subcategory: Physiological adaptation

Cognitive level: Application

---

3. A 15-year-old boy is admitted to the telemetry unit because of a suspected cardiac arrhythmia. The nurse applies five electrodes to his chest and attaches the leadwires. Identify the area where she would place the chest lead (V_1).

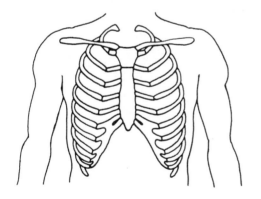

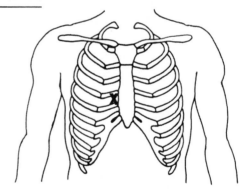

Rationale: The V_1 lead is placed in the 4th intercostal space to the right of the sternum.

Nursing process step: Implementation

Client needs category: Physiological integrity

Client needs subcategory: Reduction of risk potential

Cognitive level: Knowledge

4. A 14-year-old diagnosed with acne vulgaris asks what causes it. Which factors should the nurse identify for this client?

Select all that apply:

☐ **A.** Chocolates and sweets

☐ **B.** Increased hormone levels

☐ **C.** Growth of anaerobic bacteria

☐ **D.** Caffeine

☐ **E.** Heredity

☐ **F.** Fatty foods

ANSWER: B, C, E

Rationale: Acne vulgaris is characterized by the appearance of comedones (blackheads and whiteheads). Comedones develop for various reasons, including increased hormone levels, heredity, irritation or application of irritating substances (such as cosmetics), and growth of anaerobic bacteria. A direct relationship between acne vulgaris and consumption of chocolates, caffeine, or fatty foods hasn't been established.

Nursing process step: Implementation

Client needs category: Physiological integrity

Client needs subcategory: Physiological adaptation

Cognitive level: Application

---

5. Piaget's final stage of cognitive development involves the ability to think in abstract terms and use the scientific method to arrive at conclusions. What is the name of this stage?

_____

ANSWER: Formal operations

Rationale: According to Piaget, the formal operations stage is the final stage of cognitive development. It begins at age 12 and develops further during adolescence.

Nursing process step: Data collection

Client needs category: Health promotion and maintenance

Client needs subcategory: Growth and development through the life span

Cognitive level: Knowledge

6. Increased intake of which mineral is necessary for the rapid skeletal growth that occurs during adolescence?

ANSWER: Calcium

Rationale: Increased intake of calcium — one of the main components of bone — is necessary for rapid skeletal growth.

Nursing process step: Data collection

Client needs category: Health promotion and maintenance

Client needs subcategory: Growth and development through the life span

Cognitive level: Knowledge

---

7. Routine assessment of the adolescent should include screening for what abnormal curvature of the spine?

ANSWER: Scoliosis

Rationale: Health screening guidelines include assessing all children older than age 10 for scoliosis.

Nursing process step: Data collection

Client needs category: Health promotion and maintenance

Client needs subcategory: Growth and development through the life span

Cognitive level: Knowledge

Part 5

Psychiatric and mental health nursing

1. A client becomes angry and belligerent toward the nurse after speaking on the phone with his mother. The nurse recognizes this as what coping mechanism?

_____

ANSWER: Displacement

Rationale: Displacement is a coping mechanism in which a person transfers his feelings for one person toward another person who is less threatening.

Nursing process step: Data collection

Client needs category: Psychosocial integrity

Client needs subcategory: Psychosocial adaptation

Cognitive level: Comprehension

2. A client is presented with the treatment option of electroconvulsive therapy (ECT). After discussing the treatment with the staff, the client requests that a family member come in to help him decide whether or not to undergo this treatment. What principle does the nurse consider in supporting the client's right to self-determination and autonomy?

_____

ANSWER: Informed consent

Rationale: A client may ask for a family member's assistance in the treatment decision-making process at any time. During these times, the nurse must recognize that the client isn't ready to give informed consent.

Nursing process step: Evaluation

Client needs category: Psychosocial integrity

Client needs subcategory: Psychosocial adaptation

Cognitive level: Application

3. A female client is admitted to the emergency department (ED) after being sexually assaulted. The nurse notes that the client is sitting calmly and quietly in the examination room and recognizes this behavior as a protective defense mechanism. What defense mechanism is the client exhibiting?

_____

ANSWER: Denial

Rationale: Denial is a protective and adaptive reaction to increased anxiety. It involves consciously disowning intolerable thoughts and impulses. This response is often seen in victims of sexual abuse.

Nursing process step: Data collection

Client needs category: Psychosocial integrity

Client needs subcategory: Psychosocial adaptation

Cognitive level: Comprehension

---

4. On the second day of hospitalization, the client is discussing with the nurse concerns about unhealthy family relationships. During the nurse-client interaction, the client changes the subject to a job situation. The nurse responds, "Let's go back to what we were just talking about." What therapeutic communication technique did the nurse use?

_____

ANSWER: Focusing

Rationale: The therapeutic communication technique used by the nurse to redirect a client back to the original topic of discussion is called focusing. Focusing fosters the client's self-control and helps avoid vague generalizations, so the client can accept responsibility for facing problems.

Nursing process step: Implementation

Client needs category: Psychosocial integrity

Client needs subcategory: Psychosocial adaptation

Cognitive level: Application

5. The nurse is explaining the Bill of Rights for psychiatric patients to a client who has voluntarily sought admission to an inpatient psychiatric facility. Which of the following rights should the nurse include in the discussion?

Select all that apply:

☐ **A.** Right to select health care team members

☐ **B.** Right to refuse treatment

☐ **C.** Right to a written treatment plan

☐ **D.** Right to obtain disability

☐ **E.** Right to confidentiality

☐ **F.** Right to personal mail

ANSWER: B, C, E, F

Rationale: An inpatient client usually receives a copy of the Bill of Rights for psychiatric patients, which includes options B, C, E, and F. However, a client in an inpatient setting cannot select health team members. A client may apply for disability as a result of a chronic, incapacitating illness; however, disability is not a patient right, and members of a psychiatric institution do not decide who should receive it.

Nursing process step: Implementation

Client needs category: Psychosocial integrity

Client needs subcategory: Coping and adaptation

Cognitive level: Application

---

6. In the ED, a client reveals to the nurse a lethal plan for committing suicide and agrees to a voluntary admission to the psychiatric unit. Which information will the nurse discuss with the client to answer the question, "How long do I have to stay here?"

Select all that apply:

☐ **A.** "You may leave the hospital at any time unless you are suicidal."

☐ **B.** "Let's talk more after the health team has assessed you."

☐ **C.** "Once you've signed the papers, you have no say."

☐ **D.** "Because you could hurt yourself, you must be safe before being discharged."

☐ **E.** "You need a lawyer to help you make that decision."

☐ **F.** "There must be a court hearing before you leave the hospital."

ANSWER: A, B, D

Rationale: A person who is admitted to a psychiatric hospital on a voluntary basis may sign out of the hospital unless the health care team determines that the person is harmful to himself or others. The health care team evaluates the client's condition before discharge. If there is reason to believe that the client is harmful to himself or others, a hearing can be held to determine if the admission status should be changed from voluntary to involuntary. Option C is incorrect because it denies the client's rights; option E is incorrect because the client doesn't need a lawyer to leave the hospital; and option F is incorrect because a hearing isn't mandated before discharge. A hearing is held only if the client remains unsafe and requires further treatment.

Nursing process step: Implementation

Client needs category: Psychosocial integrity

Client needs subcategory: Coping and adaptation

Cognitive level: Application

7. The nurse has developed a relationship with a client who has an addiction problem. Which information would indicate that the therapeutic interaction is in the working stage?

Select all that apply:

☐ **A.** The client addresses how the addiction has contributed to family distress.

☐ **B.** The client reluctantly shares the family history of addiction.

☐ **C.** The client verbalizes difficulty identifying personal strengths.

☐ **D.** The client discusses the financial problems related to the addiction.

☐ **E.** The client expresses uncertainty about meeting with the nurse.

☐ **F.** The client acknowledges the addiction's effects on the children.

ANSWER: A, C, F

Rationale: Options A, C, and F are examples of the nurse-client working phase of an interaction. In the working phase, the client explores, evaluates, and determines solutions to identified problems. Options B, C, and E address what happens during the introductory phase of the nurse-client interaction.

Nursing process step: Evaluation

Client needs category: Psychosocial integrity

Client needs subcategory: Psychosocial adaptation

Cognitive level: Analysis

Anxiety disorders

1. After receiving a referral from the occupational health nurse, a client comes to the mental health clinic with a suspected diagnosis of obsessive-compulsive disorder. The client explains that his compulsion to wash his hands is interfering with his job. Which interventions are appropriate when caring for a client with this disorder?

Select all that apply:

☐ **A.** Don't allow the client time to carry out the ritualistic behavior.

☐ **B.** Support the use of appropriate defense mechanisms.

☐ **C.** Encourage the client to suppress his anxious feelings.

☐ **D.** Explore the patterns leading to the compulsive behavior.

☐ **E.** Listen attentively, but don't offer feedback.

☐ **F.** Encourage activities, such as listening to music.

ANSWER: B, D, F

Rationale: Client care should focus on reducing associated anxiety, fear, and guilt. This can be accomplished by allowing the client to carry out ritualistic behavior until he can be distracted to some other activity. The client should also be encouraged to use appropriate defense mechanisms and express his feelings of anxiety. Exploring patterns that lead to the compulsive behavior may also be effective. The nurse should always listen attentively to the client and offer feedback. Activities such as listening to music may divert the client's attention from unwanted thoughts.

Nursing process step: Implementation

Client needs category: Psychosocial integrity

Client needs subcategory: Psychosocial adaptation

Cognitive level: Application

2. After being examined by the forensic nurse in the emergency department, a rape victim is prepared for discharge. Due to the nature of the attack, this client is at risk for posttraumatic stress disorder (PTSD). Which symptoms are associated with PTSD?

Select all that apply:

☐ **A.** Recurrent, intrusive recollections or nightmares

☐ **B.** Gingival and dental problems

☐ **C.** Sleep disturbances

☐ **D.** Flight of ideas

☐ **E.** Unusual talkativeness

☐ **F.** Difficulty concentrating

ANSWER: A, C, F

Rationale: Clients diagnosed with PTSD typically experience recurrent, intrusive recollections or nightmares, sleep disturbances, difficulty concentrating, chronic anxiety or panic attacks, memory impairment, and feelings of detachment or estrangement that destroy interpersonal relationships. Gingival and dental problems are associated with bulimia. Flight of ideas and unusual talkativeness are characteristic of the acute manic phase of bipolar affective disorder.

Nursing process step: Data collection

Client needs category: Psychosocial integrity

Client needs subcategory: Psychosocial adaptation

Cognitive level: Comprehension

---

3. A physician prescribes clomipramine (Anafranil) for a client diagnosed with obsessive-compulsive disorder. What instructions should the nurse include when teaching the client about this medication?

Select all that apply:

☐ **A.** Avoid hazardous activities that require alertness or good coordination until adverse central nervous system (CNS) effects are known.

☐ **B.** Avoid alcohol and other depressants.

☐ **C.** Use saliva substitutes or sugarless candy or gum to relieve dry mouth.

☐ **D.** Take the drug on an empty stomach.

☐ **E.** Avoid using over-the-counter products, except antihistamines and decongestants, without medical permission.

☐ **F.** Discontinue the medication if adverse reactions are troublesome.

ANSWER: A, B, C

Rationale: Clomipramine, a tricyclic antidepressant used to treat obsessive-compulsive disorder, may cause adverse CNS effects. Therefore, the nurse should warn the client to avoid hazardous activities that require alertness or good coordination until its effects are known. The client should also be instructed to avoid alcohol and other depressants. Dry mouth, a common adverse effect of this medication, can be relieved with saliva substitutes or sugarless candy or gum. The nurse should tell the client to take the medication with meals (not on an empty stomach), especially during the adjustment period, to minimize adverse GI effects. Later, the entire daily dose can be taken at bedtime. The nurse should encourage the client to continue therapy, even if adverse reactions are troublesome. The client shouldn't stop taking the medication without medical permission.

Nursing process step: Implementation

Client needs category: Physiological integrity

Client needs subcategory: Pharmacological therapies

Cognitive level: Application

4. A registered nurse caring for a client with generalized anxiety disorder identifies a nursing diagnosis of *Anxiety*. The short-term goal identified is: "The client will identify his physical, emotional, and behavioral responses to anxiety." Which nursing interventions will help the client achieve this goal?

Select all that apply:

☐ **A.** Avoid talking about the client's sources of stress.

☐ **B.** Advise the client that consuming one glass of red wine per day may lessen his anxiety.

☐ **C.** Explain to the client that expressing his feelings through journal writing may increase his anxiety.

☐ **D.** Observe the client for overt signs of anxiety.

☐ **E.** Help the client connect anxiety with uncomfortable physical, emotional, or behavioral responses.

☐ **F.** Introduce the client to new strategies for coping with anxiety, such as relaxation techniques and exercise.

ANSWER: D, E, F

Rationale: The nurse should observe the client for overt signs of anxiety to assess anxiety and establish care priorities. She should also help the client connect anxiety with uncomfortable physical, emotional, or behavioral responses. To modify the automatic response to stress, the client needs to connect the anxiety experience with the unpleasant symptoms. The nurse should also introduce the client to new coping strategies, such as relaxation techniques and exercise, which can enable him to take personal responsibility for making changes. The nurse should work with the client to identify sources of stress — not avoid talking about it. The nurse should advise the client to avoid using caffeine, nicotine, and alcohol to cope with anxiety. Nicotine and caffeine are stimulants; alcohol acts as a depressant but, over time, requires increased use to achieve the desired effect, which may lead to alcohol abuse. The nurse should encourage the client to use a journal to record feelings, behaviors, stressful events, and coping strategies used to address anxiety. Documentation may help the client become aware of his anxiety and the ways in which it affects his overall functioning.

Nursing process step: Implementation

Client needs category: Psychosocial integrity

Client needs subcategory: Psychosocial adaptation

Cognitive level: Application

5. After months of coaxing by her husband, a client comes to the mental health clinic. She reports that she suffers from an overwhelming fear of leaving her house. This overwhelming fear has caused the client to lose her job and is beginning to take a toll on her marriage. What disorder would you expect the physician to diagnose?

ANSWER: Agoraphobia

Rationale: Agoraphobia is an irrational and disproportionate fear of leaving the house. In most cases, the client is aware that the fear is unreasonable or excessive. A diagnosis of agoraphobia should only be made when the avoidant behavior causes problems in occupational functioning or social relationships or if the client is distressed about having the fear.

Nursing process step: Data collection

Client needs category: Psychosocial integrity

Client needs subcategory: Psychosocial adaptation

Cognitive level: Comprehension

6. A 54-year-old client diagnosed with generalized anxiety disorder is prescribed buspirone 5 mg by mouth three times per day. In addition, the client undergoes therapy in which she's encouraged to promote relaxation by consciously controlling body functions, such as blood pressure, heart and respiratory rates, temperature, and perspiration. What's the name of the method that involves use of an electronic device to inform the client when changes in these functions occur?

_____

ANSWER: Biofeedback

Rationale: Biofeedback is a method of promoting relaxation by consciously controlling body functions, such as blood pressure, heart and respiratory rates, temperature, and perspiration. This method involves the use of an electronic device that informs the client when changes in these functions occur. Biofeedback is typically used for stress-related disorders, such as anxiety, insomnia, headaches, hypertension, asthma, GI disorders, and hyperactivity in children.

Nursing process step: Implementation

Client needs category: Psychosocial integrity

Client needs subcategory: Psychosocial adaptation

Cognitive level: Knowledge

Mood, adjustment, and dementia disorders

1. The nurse is caring for a client who talks freely about feeling depressed. During an interaction, the nurse heard the client state, "Things will never change." What other indications of hopelessness would the nurse look for?

Select all that apply:

☐ **A.** Bouts of anger

☐ **B.** Periods of irritability

☐ **C.** Preoccupation with delusions

☐ **D.** Feelings of worthlessness

☐ **E.** Self-destructive statements

☐ **F.** Intense interpersonal relationships

ANSWER: A, B, D

Rationale: Clients who are depressed and express hopelessness also tend to manifest inappropriate expressions of anger, periods of irritability, and feelings of worthlessness. Options C and F are usually seen in clients with schizophrenia; they aren't typically seen in those who express hopelessness.

Nursing process step: Data collection

Client needs category: Psychosocial integrity

Client needs subcategory: Psychosocial adaptation

Cognitive level: Analysis

2. The nurse interviews the family of a client who is hospitalized with severe depression and suicidal ideation. Which family assessment information is essential to formulating an effective plan of care?

Select all that apply:

☐ **A.** Physical pain

☐ **B.** Personal responsibilities

☐ **C.** Employment skills

☐ **D.** Communication patterns

☐ **E.** Role expectations

☐ **F.** Current family stressors

ANSWER: D, E, F

Rationale: When working with the family of a depressed client, it's helpful for the nurse to be aware of the family's communication style, the role expectations for its members, and current family stressors. This information can help to identify family difficulties and teaching points that could benefit the client and the family. Information concerning physical pain, personal responsibilities, and employment skills wouldn't be helpful because these areas aren't directly related to their experience of having a depressed family member.

Nursing process step: Planning

Client needs category: Psychosocial integrity

Client needs subcategory: Psychosocial adaptation

Cognitive level: Analysis

---

3. A client is prescribed sertraline (Zoloft), a selective serotonin reuptake inhibitor. Which information about this drug's adverse effects would the nurse include when creating a medication teaching plan?

Select all that apply:

☐ **A.** Agitation

☐ **B.** Agranulocytosis

☐ **C.** Sleep disturbance

☐ **D.** Intermittent tachycardia

☐ **E.** Dry mouth

☐ **F.** Seizures

ANSWER: A, C, E

Rationale: Common adverse effects of Zoloft include agitation, sleep disturbance, and dry mouth. Agranulocytosis, intermittent tachycardia, and seizures are adverse effects of clozapine (Clozaril).

Nursing process step: Planning

Client needs category: Physiological integrity

Client needs subcategory: Pharmacological therapies

Cognitive level: Knowledge

4. The nurse is assessing a client to determine whether he is suffering from dementia or depression. Which information helps the nurse to differentiate between the two?

Select all that apply:

☐ **A.** The progression of symptoms is slow.

☐ **B.** The client answers questions with, "I don't know."

☐ **C.** The client acts apathetic and pessimistic.

☐ **D.** The family can't identify when the symptoms first appeared.

☐ **E.** The client's basic personality has changed.

☐ **F.** The client has great difficulty paying attention to others.

ANSWER: A, D, E, F

Rationale: Common characteristics of dementia include a slow onset of symptoms, difficulty identifying when the symptoms first occurred, noticeable changes in the client's personality, and impaired ability to pay attention to other people. Options B and C are symptoms of depression, not dementia.

Nursing process step: Data collection

Client needs category: Psychosocial integrity

Client needs subcategory: Coping and adaptation

Cognitive level: Analysis

5. A client has been diagnosed with an adjustment disorder of mixed anxiety and depression. Which of the following nursing diagnoses are associated with a client who has an adjustment disorder?

Select all that apply:

☐ **A.** Activity intolerance

☐ **B.** Impaired social interaction

☐ **C.** Self-esteem disturbance

☐ **D.** Personal identity disturbance

☐ **E.** Acute confusion

☐ **F.** Impaired memory

ANSWER: B AND C

Rationale: A client with an adjustment disorder is likely to have impaired social interaction and self-esteem disturbance. The other nursing diagnoses aren't related to the diagnosis of adjustment disorder.

Nursing process step: Data collection

Client needs category: Psychosocial integrity

Client needs subcategory: Psychosocial adaptation

Cognitive level: Analysis

1. A physician prescribes lithium for a client diagnosed with bipolar disorder. The nurse needs to provide appropriate education for the client on this drug. Which of the following topics should the nurse cover?

Select all that apply:

☐ **A.** The potential for addiction

☐ **B.** Signs and symptoms of drug toxicity

☐ **C.** The potential for tardive dyskinesia

☐ **D.** A low-tyramine diet

☐ **E.** The need to consistently monitor blood levels

☐ **F.** Changes in his mood that may take 7 to 21 days

ANSWER: B, E, F

Rationale: Client education should cover the signs and symptoms of drug toxicity as well as the need to report them to the physician. The client should be instructed to monitor his lithium levels on a regular basis to avoid toxicity. The nurse should explain that 7 to 21 days may pass before the client notes a change in his mood. Lithium does not have addictive properties. Tyramine is a potential concern to clients taking monoamine-oxidase inhibitors.

Nursing process step: Implementation

Client needs category: Physiological integrity

Client needs subcategory: Pharmacological therapies

Cognitive level: Application

---

2. The nurse is monitoring a client who appears to be hallucinating. She notes paranoid content in the client's speech and he appears agitated. The client is gesturing at a figure on the television. Which of the following nursing interventions are appropriate?

Select all that apply:

☐ **A.** In a firm voice, instruct the client to stop the behavior.

☐ **B.** Reinforce that the client is not in any danger.

☐ **C.** Acknowledge the presence of the hallucinations.

☐ **D.** Instruct other team members to ignore the client's behavior.

☐ **E.** Immediately implement physical restraint procedures.

☐ **F.** Use a calm voice and simple commands.

ANSWER: B, C, F

Rationale: Using a calm voice, the nurse should reassure the client that he is safe. She shouldn't challenge the client; rather, she should acknowledge his hallucinatory experience. It is not appropriate to request that the client stop the behavior. Implementing restraints is not warranted at this time. Although the client is agitated, no evidence exists that the client is at risk for harming himself or others.

Nursing process step: Implementation

Client needs category: Psychosocial integrity

Client needs subcategory: Psychosocial adaptation

Cognitive level: Application

3. A client with schizophrenia is taking the atypical antipsychotic medication clozapine (Clozaril). Which of the following signs and symptoms indicate the presence of adverse effects associated with this medication?

Select all that apply:

☐ **A.** Sore throat

☐ **B.** Pill-rolling movements

☐ **C.** Polyuria

☐ **D.** Fever

☐ **E.** Polydipsia

☐ **F.** Orthostatic hypotension

ANSWER: A, D

Rationale: Sore throat, fever, and sudden onset of other flulike symptoms are signs of agranulocytosis. The condition is caused by a lack of a sufficient number of granulocytes (a type of white blood cell), which causes the individual to be susceptible to infection. The client's white blood cell count should be monitored at least weekly throughout the course of treatment. Pill-rolling movements can occur in those experiencing extrapyramidal adverse effects associated with antipsychotic medication that has been prescribed for much longer than a medication such as clozapine. Polydipsia (excessive thirst) and polyuria (increased urine) are common adverse effects of lithium. Orthostatic hypotension is an adverse effect of tricyclic antidepressants.

Nursing process step: Data collection

Client needs category: Physiological integrity

Client needs subcategory: Pharmacological therapies

Cognitive level: Application

---

4. A delusional client approaches the nurse, stating, "I am the Easter bunny," and insisting that the nurse refer to him as such. The belief appears to be fixed and unchanging. Which of the following nursing interventions should the nurse implement when working with this client?

Select all that apply:

☐ **A.** Consistently use the client's name in interaction.

☐ **B.** Smile at the humor of the situation.

☐ **C.** Agree that the client is the Easter Bunny.

☐ **D.** Logically point out why the client could not be the Easter Bunny.

☐ **E.** Provide an as-needed medication.

☐ **F.** Provide the client with structured activities.

ANSWER: A, F

Rationale: Continued reality-based orientation is necessary, so it is appropriate to use the client's name in any interaction. Structured activities can help the client refocus and resolve his delusion. The nurse shouldn't contribute to the delusion by going along with the situation or smiling at the humor of the circumstances. Logical arguments and an as-needed medication aren't likely to change the client's beliefs.

Nursing process step: Implementation

Client needs category: Psychosocial integrity

Client needs subcategory: Coping and adaptation

Cognitive level: Analysis

5. A physician starts a client on the antipsychotic medication haloperidol (Haldol). The nurse is aware that this medication has extrapyramidal adverse effects. Which of the following measures should the nurse take during Haldol administration?

Select all that apply:

☐ **A.** Review subcutaneous injection technique.

☐ **B.** Closely monitor vital signs, especially temperature.

☐ **C.** Provide the client with the opportunity to pace.

☐ **D.** Monitor blood glucose levels.

☐ **E.** Provide the client with hard candy.

☐ **F.** Monitor for signs and symptoms of urticaria.

ANSWER: B, C, E

Rationale: Neuroleptic malignant syndrome is a life-threatening extrapyramidal adverse effect of antipsychotic medications such as Haldol. It's associated with a rapid increase in temperature. The most common extrapyramidal adverse effect, akathisia, is a form of psychomotor restlessness that can often be relieved by pacing. Haldol and the anticholinergic medications that are provided to alleviate its extrapyramidal effects can result in dry mouth. Providing the client with hard candy to suck on can help alleviate this problem. Haldol isn't given subcutaneously and doesn't affect blood glucose levels. Urticaria is not usually associated with Haldol administration.

Nursing process step: Planning

Client needs category: Physiological integrity

Client needs subcategory: Pharmacological therapies

Cognitive level: Analysis

---

6. The nurse observes that a client diagnosed with schizophrenia is staring into space and doesn't acknowledge the presence of others. At times, the client moves rapidly but then stops and remains in one posture for long periods. What form of schizophrenia is the nurse observing?

ANSWER: Catatonic

Rationale: A client with catatonic schizophrenia shows a lack of responsiveness to the environment. The client may move rapidly or slowly, often alternating between patterns of movement. In many cases, he then poses and appears rigid. The other forms of schizophrenia — paranoid, disorganized, undifferentiated, and residual — are associated with different patterns of behavior and responses. However, disruption of motor behavior in conjunction with a lack of responsiveness to the immediate environment occurs only in the catatonic form of schizophrenia.

Nursing process step: Data collection

Client needs category: Psychosocial integrity

Client needs subcategory: Psychosocial adaptation

Cognitive level: Knowledge

7. A client with schizophrenia displays a lack of interest in activities, reduced affect, and poor ability to perform activities of daily living (ADLs). What term would be used to describe this clustering of symptoms?

_____

ANSWER: Negative

Rationale: Schizophrenic clients often display positive and negative symptoms. Negative symptoms are characterized by the absence of typically displayed emotional responses. Clients with these symptoms tend to respond poorly to medication. Positive symptoms, such as auditory or visual hallucinations, are characterized by enhancement of a sensory modality.

Nursing process step: Data collection

Client needs category: Psychosocial integrity

Client needs subcategory: Psychosocial adaptation

Cognitive level: Knowledge

---

8. One of the causes of schizophrenia involves an overstimulation of what neurotransmitter?

_____

ANSWER: Dopamine

Rationale: Studies on the role of neurotransmitters in schizophrenia have identified that the disease results (at least in part) from an overactive dopamine system in the brain. Excessive dopamine activity may be responsible for such symptoms as hallucinations, agitation, delusional thinking, and grandiosity — forms of hyperactivity that have been linked to excessive dopamine activity.

Nursing process step: Data collection

Client needs category: Physiological integrity

Client needs subcategory: Physiological adaptation

Cognitive level: Knowledge

Substance abuse, eating disorders, and impulse control disorders

1. An adolescent client is being admitted to the psychiatric unit for treatment of an eating disorder. Her admission interview reveals a history of recurrent episodes of binge eating and self-induced vomiting. The nurse recognizes these as symptoms of what disease?

_____

Answer: Bulimia nervosa

Rationale: The essential features of bulimia nervosa include eating binges followed by feelings of guilt, humiliation, and self-deprecation. These feelings cause the client to engage in self-induced vomiting, use laxatives or diuretics, follow a strict diet, or fast to overcome the effects of the binges.

Nursing process step: Data collection

Client needs category: Psychosocial integrity

Client needs subcategory: Psychosocial adaptation

Cognitive level: Knowledge

2. While the nurse is collecting data on a client who has a history of multiple substance abuse, the client reports that he's experiencing nausea, vomiting, and diarrhea. The nurse observes flushing, piloerection, increased lacrimation, and rhinorrhea. These symptoms probably indicate withdrawal from what category of drugs?

_____

Answer: Opioid

Rationale: Typical symptoms of opioid addiction and withdrawal include flushing, piloerection, nausea, vomiting, abdominal cramps, increased lacrimation, and rhinorrhea. The nurse must be alert for these withdrawal symptoms because of increased abuse of opioids, such as heroine and hydrocodone.

Nursing process step: Data collection

Client needs category: Psychosocial integrity

Client needs subcategory: Psychosocial adaptation

Cognitive level: Knowledge

3. The nurse is assisting in the discharge planning for a client with alcoholism. What outpatient support group should she refer the client to?

_____

ANSWER: Alcoholics Anonymous

Rationale: Alcoholics Anonymous is an outpatient support group that allows clients to share their problems related to alcohol abuse and gain support from group members to avoid further abuse.

Nursing process step: Planning

Client needs category: Safe, effective care environment

Client needs subcategory: Coordinated care

Cognitive level: Analysis

---

4. Which of the following interventions would be supportive for a client with a nursing diagnosis of imbalanced nutrition — consuming less than the body requires due to dysfunctional eating patterns?

Select all that apply:

☐ **A.** Provide small, frequent feedings.

☐ **B.** Monitor weight gain.

☐ **C.** Allow the client to skip meals until the antidepressant levels are therapeutic.

☐ **D.** Encourage journaling to promote the expression of feelings.

☐ **E.** Monitor the client at mealtimes and for an hour after meals.

☐ **F.** Encourage the client to eat three substantial meals a day.

ANSWER: A, B, D, E

Rationale: Smaller meals may be better tolerated by the client and will gradually increase her daily caloric intake. The nurse should monitor the client's weight because an anorexic will hide weight loss. Anorexics are emotionally restrained and afraid of their feelings, so journaling can be a powerful tool that assists in recovery. Anorexic clients are obsessed with gaining weight and will skip all meals if given the opportunity. Because of self-starvation, they seldom can tolerate large meals three times a day.

Nursing process step: Implementation

Client needs category: Psychosocial integrity

Client needs subcategory: Psychosocial adaptation

Cognitive level: Analysis

5. While collecting data on a client who was diagnosed with impulse control disorder (and who displays violent, aggressive, and assaultive behavior), the nurse can expect to find which of the following assessments?

Select all that apply:

☐ **A.** The client functions well in other areas of his life.

☐ **B.** The degree of aggressiveness is out of proportion to the stressor.

☐ **C.** The client often uses a stressor to justify the violent behavior.

☐ **D.** The client has a history of parental alcoholism and a chaotic, abusive family life.

☐ **E.** The client shows no remorse about his inability to control his behavior.

Rationale: A client with an impulse control disorder who displays violent, aggressive, and assaultive behavior generally functions well in other areas of his life. The degree of the client's aggressiveness is disproportionate to the stressor, and the client commonly has a history of parental alcoholism, as well as a chaotic family life. The client often verbalizes sincere guilt and remorse for the aggressive behavior.

Nursing process step: Data collection

Client needs category: Psychosocial integrity

Client needs subcategory: Psychosocial adaptation

Cognitive level: Application